Diving In

Discovering Who You Are
in the Second Half of Life

MARK BODNARCZUK

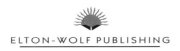

ELTON-WOLF PUBLISHING

Diving In

Discovering Who You Are in the Second Half of Life

Text edited by Cliff Carle

Cover design by David Marty

Text design by Monica Nieman

Published by Elton-Wolf Publishing

Seattle, Washington

ISBN: 1-58619-045-8

Library of Congress Catalog Number: 2003102512

07 06 05 04 03   1 2 3 4 5

First Edition April 2003

Printed in Canada

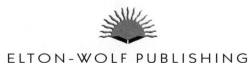

ELTON-WOLF PUBLISHING

2505 Second Avenue Suite 515 Seattle, Washington 98121
Tel 206.748.0345 Fax 206.748.0343
www.elton-wolf.com info@elton-wolf.com
Seattle • Los Angeles

FOR MY BELOVED FAMILY

For Elin my wife who loves me, and grounds me in the pleasures and realities of life and who supports me in my passion for diving and exploring the inner life.

For my stepdaughter Juliana who has been a facilitator of deep personal change in my life and has taught me about valuing the differences in others.

For my son Thomas who has given me a renewed sense of meaning, purpose, and long-term responsibility in my life.

ACKNOWLEDGMENTS

It was Anne Avery, Jungian analyst and friend, who guided me on my eighteen-year journey of inner diving into the unfathomable depths of the unconscious. She taught me that every analyst's or therapist's goal should be to work themselves out of a job by teaching their clients how to carry on the process of psychological growth for themselves.

Don Richard Riso and Russ Hudson trained me in the Enneagram and they remain mentors and friends. Don's depth of person, transparency of self, passion for psychological truth, and articulation of the wisdom of the Enneagram have made an enormous difference in my life and the lives of my family, friends, and clients.

Much of the diving element of this book came from my trip aboard the Peter Hughes Diving boat, the Komodo Dancer. I would like to thank Peter Hughes for giving me permission to use my picture of the Komodo Dancer on the front cover. I would also like to thank the crew, especially Gary Bevan, Susanna Hinderks, and Yan Alfian who were my underwater guides and diving companions during the trip. Ronald de Boer and Guido Brink were my buddies on many a dive. Guido and I talked about philosophy and psychology, and did an unforgettable blue water dive where a group of enormous manta rays appeared from the bottomless abyss of the ocean floor that was a thousand feet beneath us.

In terms of the writing and production of the book, I would like to offer special thanks to Frank Hawkins, one of my closest friends and a mentor, who was always willing to review and discuss my ideas and machinations.

Lee Synnott was enormously helpful with feedback on an earlier draft of the book, and instrumental in steering me in the right direction in the publishing world.

My friend Joe Pries was the inspiration for me to "Just tell a story," a comment that haunted me, and helped spark the idea for the form the current book has taken.

Thanks to Jim McIntyre who gave me valuable input from the perspective of a professional scuba instructor.

To Anthony Malensek, business partner and long-time friend who has helped in the production of this book in more ways than I can explain.

Finally, I would also like to thank the people who took countless hours to review an earlier draft, and whose input caused me to rewrite the book in its entirety. This resulted in a much better product: Jonathan Babicz, Michael Brandt, Simon Caruthers, Carol Cilona, Annie Fox, Bob Gorab, Sue Gruber, Bill Jackson, Lynn Kaemmerer, Greg Kobliska, Elin Larson, Sue Locke, Larry Lunceford, Melissa Matsuura, Tom Neils, Tom Prosapio, Neil Redman, Marvin Shear, Cathy Staton, Carrie Sterns, Dennis Tallon, and Nancy Weidenfeller.

CONTENTS

LIST OF FIGURES

INTRODUCTION

Scuba diving has long been used as a metaphor for inner, psychic exploration. People like the psychiatrist Carl Jung have been likened to scuba divers who have mapped out the uncharted depths of the human personality below the surface waters of consciousness. But to my knowledge, none of the people who use this metaphor are actually scuba divers. Some years ago when I began diving, my eighteen years of inner exploration with a Jungian analyst, and the power and majesty of the underwater world, merged into an artesian passion that welled up from the depths of my soul. As a *scuba diver*, I became a kind of amphibian where my dive gear allowed me to live temporarily in a world that was in between land and sea. As an *inner diver* I became a kind of amphibian who used the competencies described in this book to explore the relationship between the pedestrian questions that linger on the surface of life, and the existential questions of ultimate meaning that lurk beneath the surface of consciousness.

My desire to explore the underwater ocean world led me to travel to places like Hawaii, Indonesia, Australia, Fiji, Palau, Egypt, and Bikini Atoll in the Marshall Islands. My desire to explore the uncharted depths of my own personality led me beyond the insights I internalized from Jung to a personality typology called the Enneagram. I found that the nine Enneagram types were one of the most powerful descriptions of human behavior and motivation that I had ever encountered. Not only did the nine types describe and predict people's behavior, they also laid bare many of the motives that drove these behaviors.

For a number of years, my Jungian and Enneagram views ran on separate tracks. I found myself teaching and using them side-by-side with no elegant way to integrate the *empirical* power of the Enneagram to describe and predict people's motives and behavior, with the *theoretical* power of a model of personality I had developed that echoed Jung's work, but was not strictly speaking Jungian.

When the outlines of a synthesis between my own post-Jungian view and the Enneagram began to emerge into a new model of the human personality, I decided to write a book that described the synthesis. The feedback that I received from readers of earlier drafts of this book brutally hammered home the fact that it read too much like a college textbook. Luckily for me, one reviewer exclaimed in exasperation, "Just tell a story!" A few weeks later, as I flew high above the South China Sea on my way to embark on an eleven-day dive trip in Indonesia aboard the dive ship Komodo Dancer, these words, "Just tell a story," haunted me, so that's what I decided to do. I turned my attention to the task of rewriting the book as a *teaching novel* that explores the metaphoric connections between scuba diving, the Enneagram, and my model for exploring the hidden realms of the human personality as an inner diver. *Diving In: Discovering Who You Are in the Second Half of Life*, became both a story and a psychological process that is described in the teaching sessions of the dive workshop.

As a story, *Diving In* is about scuba diving, adventure, and the lives of people who are in pursuit of deep personal change. It is about nine people who are real, but whose identities have been changed, so, to coin a phrase, the book is *real fiction*. I chose these nine people because they powerfully exemplified the nine Enneagram types. Parts of their story will be your story, or the story of people you know. So, while some knowledge of the Enneagram is helpful, it is not necessary. Nonetheless, I have included a brief summary of the nine types in the back of this book.[1] This cast of nine attends a dive workshop on the 110-foot sailing vessel *Explorer* in Indonesia that totally removes them from the context of their everyday lives. Three times a day, they learn about the depths of their personality in one-hour sessions held around an enormous wooden teaching table on the main deck of a ship that is floating in the middle of nowhere. Each teaching session is followed by a one-hour reflective time of diving where they view the spectacular coral reefs and undersea life of Indonesia from Bali to Komodo Island, and hear nothing under-water but the sound of air bubbles.

The teaching sessions of the book describe the path of *Discovering Who You Are in the Second Half of Life* as a natural process of psychological growth that happens to all people, in all times, in all places. It is similar to what Jung called the process of Individuation. The awareness of the calling to discover who we really are becomes more pronounced as people approach the second half of life, as is the case with the nine people in this story. Each of them has spent the first half of their lives running the race to construct a life and a self. As they approach the second half of life, each one runs smack into a brick wall of either outer crisis and pressure in their day-to-day lives, or the inner crisis and pressure to discover their destiny and unique purpose in life.

Whether you are a scuba diver who enjoys diving in exotic places; a person in the second half of life searching for your destiny and a sense of meaning in life; a student or teacher of the Enneagram looking for connections to new psychological traditions;

someone of any age who is tired of the quick fix, band-aid approach of most self-help books; or a therapist or Jungian analyst searching for new psychological models to use with your clients, come along on the dive ship *Explorer* and see which of the people decide to answer their calling to deep personal change by *Diving In*, and which ones check out before the workshop ends.

Beginning the Journey

THE HIGH CHAIR TYRANT

"Lock the door!" Dan Wright barked to the managers seated in his conference room. One of them got up to carry out his command as he bellowed, "That will teach the others to be late to my meetings.

"Let's get going—we have a long agenda for today. To begin with, do any of you have any input on my latest plan for cutting overhead costs?" People stared down at the table and no one spoke up. Sally, who was new to the company, raised her hand and began presenting her views on the strengths and weaknesses of the approach. Dan placated Sally while she was reviewing the strengths of the plan, but when she actually dared to identify weaknesses, he erupted in a rage, pounded his fist on the table and screamed, "You don't know what you're talking about, woman!" He quickly moved on to the next agenda item. Dan was using a coping strategy that might have been appropriate when he was two years old. But as a fifty-year-old man and president of the SciTech Corporation, Dan Wright was acting like a *high chair tyrant*.

Everyone just looked on in silence. Now Sally knew why no one else volunteered to give him any feedback. As she left the meeting, she wanted to discuss Dan's outburst with some of her colleagues in the hope of finding some moral support, but most of them acted as if nothing had happened. When she pressed them for some feedback on what she thought was inappropriate behavior on Dan's part, they kind of sympathized with her, then moved on to another topic as quickly as possible, just as Dan did in the meeting. Dan's managers were well trained in the organizational culture at SciTech.

Dan Wright had a shiny, clean, well-scrubbed Ivy League look about him—with every hair in place, no one ever saw him without a dress shirt and tie on. He had always been a perfectionist who had a hard time just loosening up and having fun. From the time he was a child, Dan got a loud and clear message that mistakes would not be tolerated. His father, Jake, was a strict authoritarian who hammered into Dan's senses the edict that he was only good when he did what was right, and what was right was defined exclusively by his father's standards and measuring sticks. Because Dan had to constantly struggle with his propensity to veer off course in doing the right thing, Dan harbored the secret belief that he was somehow corrupt or defective, flawed in character.

Dan and his wife Susan met Cindy Reeder in graduate school at MIT where he finished an undergraduate degree in physics, and went straight into an MS program in electrical engineering. Cindy was a graduate assistant finishing up her Ph.D. Susan remembers the days in Cambridge fondly. The university world was an easy place to make friends because everyone had such a common focus. They were young, without children, and would travel and enjoy life on school breaks. Susan remembered dinner parties, holiday celebrations, and even bold, daring, and exotic trips, such as when Cindy, Dan and she went scuba diving in the Red Sea during the mid-1970s while Israel was still occupying the Sinai.

When Dan was not being inwardly hammered by his fixation about perfection, he displayed a deep and abiding sense of conscientiousness and an objective sense of right and wrong even in situations that were difficult for most people to figure out. But once Dan got up on his self-righteous high horse, he became rigid and intolerant of others. He went out of his way to point out and try to correct the flaws he saw in people, even in areas that were none of his business and over their protests for him to leave them alone.

After graduate school, Cindy stayed on in Cambridge to finish her degree. Cindy always liked the creative stimulation of the university and decided to take a post doc at Harvard rather than go into the frenetic world of business. Dan landed a good job in Connecticut with a company that was a defense contractor doing work at the Navy base in Groton. Dan was a careful, conservative, and insightful engineer who always did quality work, and quickly established himself as a team leader and then became a regional manager for the West Coast division of the company. Dan passed through a lot of airports traveling a hundred days a year, and was always interested in the metal detectors and X-ray scanning equipment because they related to some of the work that he was doing for the Navy.

Dan began wondering if he could produce more cost-effective, high-resolution airport X-ray equipment that would be more computer-automated, and would remove more human error in scanning baggage. He had the seed money to start a company and a three-car garage behind his house he could use as an office and fabrication facility. But he wasn't sure if the current technology could really support his idea. He drove to Cambridge to meet with Cindy, who had just accepted a position at MIT as an assistant professor. After passing the feasibility test with Cindy, Dan wrote a business plan for what became the SciTech Corporation. He secured a loan from a bank in Boston, hired Cindy as his first employee, and set about the task of hammering their ideas into a technology that could be packaged, produced, and sold to airports around the world.

Dan was obsessed with cleanliness at home and at work. He would never allow anyone to eat in his car and he was neurotic about washing it even in the winter when the trip home from the car wash alone would dirty it again. Dan would even wash rental cars before he returned them. It was almost as if the outer, compulsive, ritual washings were a metaphorical attempt to remove his own deep and abiding sense of being unclean, dirty, tarnished, and fundamentally flawed. Dan was also compulsive about orderliness, and having everything in its place, almost as though external order was a way to control the chaos he sensed deep within.

The company grew to the point where, after two years, Dan had purchased some land and broken ground on a ten thousand-square foot facility, which could expand to fifty thousand if continued business growth required it. Revenues continued the typical pattern of rising then leveling off, but after ten years the company had seventy-five employees and was generating gross revenues of over $100 million per year. The grueling development years had taken their toll on Dan both professionally and in his family life. He was feeling like he had to push harder and harder as the business grew just to get people to toe the line of quality and service that he demanded. He worked sixty to seventy hours a week and felt as if he had the world on his shoulders. But if he were to cut back, who would fill the gap?

Those who knew him best, like Cindy Reeder, had seen Dan's own duplicity, where he would follow his inner convictions about what was right and wrong to the point where he set a standard so high that even he could not keep it. Once Dan was confronted by the fact that he had violated his own standards, he would spiral down into a state of guilt, shame, self-reproach, and depression or become erratic in his behavior, moving on to another issue just to escape the condemnation.

Dan had always lived with this darker side of his personality, but he always had enough psychological energy to "manage" it and keep it under control. In a less overt way, Dan siphoned off his anger against himself and the imperfections of life by constant faultfinding, nit picking, and commenting only on the one out of a hundred things that was not done correctly. When Dan felt justified (which was most of the time), there was nothing that could stop the storm of relentless criticism and chastising that followed. Dan once hired a consultant in New York. While finalizing the scope of work, he called the consultant and emphatically told her to correct the letter of agreement. He insisted that he wanted the date on the letter to match the date on the fax. "Sure," the consultant replied. After an uncomfortable period of silence, Dan said, "This is why my people hate me, isn't it?" The consultant didn't respond because she knew better.

The pressure and drive that Dan poured into the company took its toll on his marriage to Susan, who worked part time at SciTech. Susan was pressuring Dan to sell the condo that they had at the lake and buy a larger town home to accommodate the overnight company who came to stay with them. On paper, it seemed like a good investment, but Dan was somehow bothered by her uncharacteristically demanding attitude and didn't know exactly why. Somewhere on the fringe of his consciousness a thought crept into his mind that she was planning to leave him and would use the town home as her new place of refuge. Susan remembered with longing a brief time of autonomy that she had, before meeting Dan, when she lived on her own in Toledo, Ohio. Other than this brief time, Susan had gone from the family she was raised in to being married to Dan, and never had any time to find out who she was or what she wanted in life. She always regretted not taking more time to sort this out. Had she done this, maybe she never would have married Dan in the first place.

Dan tried at all costs to avoid any experience of being wrong. One of the most difficult challenges for him was to keep his anger and rage concealed from people outside the inner circle of his friends and family. He even tried to hide it from himself. His disgust with the imperfections of his staff, and of life itself, was like a pressure cooker ready to blow. Dan would show this mean side of himself to his staff and his family because he knew they would take it. At work, he threw temper tantrums, pounding his desk and demanding that things be done his way, immediately. At home, Dan and Susan's marriage was littered with broken dishes, slammed doors, and meals that had gone uneaten because Dan had stormed out of the house.

Susan was thrown into a predicament where she didn't necessarily want to break up her marriage, but she wanted to find the autonomous self that she had only gotten a glimmer of many years ago. In order to support Dan financially in his studies at MIT, she had not gone to college, so to leave her marriage would be an enormous step backward in terms of her lifestyle. She had talked to Dan indirectly about her dissatisfaction with their marriage over the years, but he never seemed to take her cues. Because he would probably take the brunt of the blame for the failed marriage on himself and react with rage, Susan had given up on him actually listening to her about her concerns. Instead, things went along as they always had, and Susan would just sweep the problems out of her consciousness and under the carpet.

Dan was a hard-driving person at all times, but he was hardest on his line managers, for whom he had a zero tolerance for rework situations, quality problems, and lack of response to customer suggestions for improvement. Dan expected his managers to stay on top of the finest details of their operation. But when Dan came around looking for a real-time status report on how things were going, he totally undermined his managers' authority. One manager who Dan had embarrassed numerous times liked to sardonically joke that Dan was not a micro-manager, he was a nano-manager and a pico-manager. Some people are dead wrong, but Dan was almost always dead right because he made himself wrong through his harsh delivery and caustic style, even when he began by being right in the first place.

Dan's father, Jake, died in September 2000, after a protracted fight with cancer. Dan was actually relieved by Jake's death because the long illness had financially and psychologically drained him and Susan. But more than this, Dan had been so verbally and emotionally abused by his father's harsh, critical spirit that the death came as a relief and sense of freedom that he could not quite understand or explain. He hated his father with a passion and made a lifetime effort of avoiding every aspect of his father's style and mannerisms. Yet somehow these Herculean efforts to avoid being like his father only backfired, and Dan had slowly become a caricature of the person he so thoroughly hated.

The external pressure of running the business, along with his family issues, had worn Dan down to the point where he was beginning to wonder about how he could get out of the business and move on to doing other less stressful things. Dan didn't want to sell SciTech to an outsider because a few of his employees, like Cindy Reeder, had become friends over the years and for their sakes he was afraid of losing total control of the company. He thought about an employee buy-out plan where he could issue stock and those employees who were able could purchase a portion of the corporation, but both his lawyer and accountant had advised him against this. From his perspective, the best case scenario would have his daughter, Carol, take over the business and keep him in the loop on major decisions.

Unfortunately, his relationship with Carol had been problematic for years. Dan was a tough-minded, critical engineer and was unable to stop using this pattern of behavior when he came home from the office, even when Carol was a little girl. As she grew into her teen years, nothing was ever good enough for Dan. He would look at a math test Carol brought home, on which she scored 96 percent, and Dan would comment only on the problems she'd missed. Years later, while she was at Bucknell University studying math, Dan and Susan would visit periodically, but Dan's simmering rage about her not doing things "his way" always strained the visits. On some occasions, Dan would storm off, and insist that Susan leave Carol and follow him home.

As Carol got older she would try to argue it out with her dad, but arguing with Dan was normally a useless exercise. He was a my-way-or-the-highway kind of guy, not so much because he wanted to have power over people, but because he just knew that he was right. Once he had made up his mind about something, there was little room for discussion. Even if he did concede and do it the other person's way, Dan would do it against his will, and when things went the way he had predicted they would, he was always ready to tell people, "I told you so."

Carol had worked at SciTech part-time while she was finishing her graduate degree in computer science at Yale, and even the little interaction that she and Dan had caused nothing but friction. Over Dan's objections, she had just accepted a job with Prodigal, a software company in Washington D.C., and would be moving in a few weeks. She was happily looking to relocate so she could start her new job and move further away from the control and endless criticism of her father. He was angered and resentful that she was not staying to help him run the company, because *he* was convinced that this was the right thing for her to do.

With the coming and passing of September 11, 2001, SciTech's business more than doubled as even the smallest airports began buying and installing the most sophisticated baggage screening equipment they could find. SciTech was the top of the line in terms of technology, but was more affordable long-term than even less sophisticated screening packages.

Dan had mixed feelings about this boom in business. First, he was glad the company was financially solvent and had bright prospects for the future. But in Dan's mind, his psychological clock was ticking and it was high time for him to get out of SciTech. With each passing day he was feeling more and more trapped by his own success. With the departure of Carol, his last hope for moving in another direction in his life without totally having to give up control of the company went out the window. His resentment continued to grow toward her and toward his employees because he felt that his loyalty to them was forcing him to keep running the company. His resentment toward himself was also growing because he wasn't smart enough to figure his way out of this mess.

THE DIVE WORKSHOP

Cindy Reeder would be one person that Dan could trust to take over the company, but she doesn't want it. She is perfectly happy as Director of R&D, thinking about new ideas, new technologies. Being Director of R&D is a perfect blend of the corporate world and the academic world she longs to stay connected to.

Cindy is a long-time friend of the family, back to the MIT days, and has become friends with Carol, who sits near her department. Cindy can see how toxic the relationship is between Carol and Dan at work. Carol has been confiding in Cindy that her Mom is getting ready to leave Dan, and move up to their summer home at the lake until the divorce is final. Susan has also told Cindy of her plans. Because she has been told about the impending divorce in confidence, Cindy cannot breath a word of it to Dan, her boss and long-time friend. Susan has threatened to leave Dan before, but this time her words have a tone of determination in them that Cindy has never heard before.

Unlike Dan, who hasn't been diving in years because he actually prides himself in never taking any time off, Cindy has continued to dive about twenty-five tanks a year, every year since they dove in Egypt. Cindy has just returned from a one-week live-aboard dive workshop in Indonesia. She stops by Dan's office on Monday morning just to touch base.

"How was your trip?" Dan asks, glad to see her back. "Did you learn a lot more about diving?"

"Yes," Cindy says, plopping down with a satisfied sigh in the chair next to his desk. "But I learned a lot more about myself," she says, hoping to pique his interest.

"What do you mean?" he asks.

"Well, it was a workshop on discovering who you are in the second half of life."

"Don't tell me you're going through a mid-life crisis." Dan says, only half in jest.

"It was an adventure," she replies. "The setting, on a boat in Indonesia, was purposely remote so that it totally takes you away from the context of your life—no phones, no e-mail, no nothing. It gave me a new perspective by helping me step outside of the day-to-day press of my life. The workshop was like an Outward Bound trip and involved intense teaching sessions interspersed with some of the most magnificent diving in the world. The boat becomes a kind of laboratory of human nature as you learn about yourself by interacting with others, learning new material and then taking time to reflect when you're underwater. It was incredible, just incredible, even better than the Red Sea back in the seventies."

Dan can tell where Cindy is going with her energetic description of the workshop and he tries to move on to another topic. After a few failed attempts to make her point subtly, Cindy comes right out and says, "Dan, I think you need to go on this trip."

Cindy and Dan are almost polar opposites, but somehow they have found a synergy between them by acknowledging and learning to value these differences. On the rare occasion Dan talks to anyone about what's bothering him, he talks to Cindy. He has always trusted her technical knowledge and on the personal front, Cindy has always been a facilitator of change who helped him look below the surface of things, and to see himself as he otherwise could not.

Dan is now pacing his office looking for reasons to squirm out of going on the trip. But Cindy is pressuring him in a way that is not typical, because she knows what Dan doesn't about Susan planning to leave. "I'm worried about you," Cindy says. "Watching your life is like watching an accident that's about to happen. You're heading for a wall at eighty miles an hour and you're not letting off the gas pedal."

"Look," Dan says, trying to justify not going, "you know I can't get away with my schedule, besides my wife complains that I'm never home to help around the house."

"I don't think Susan would mind if you went," Cindy counters, "she would probably be in favor of it. Besides, Dan, I'm really worried about you."

This open and deep display of feelings and care has him wavering. He knows Cindy is his friend, is being sincere, and has no ulterior motive behind her empathy. "I haven't dove for over three years," Dan says, beginning to soften.

"Don't worry, Dan," she assures him, "the trip is designed for people at all diving levels. Many of the dive sites are in sheltered harbors, and the crew reads the tides really well so the currents are very manageable."

The phone rings, and Dan's off and running, thrown into the first of a myriad of problems that typically drive his day at a frenetic pace. Cindy waves, as he talks on and acknowledges her leaving in passing.

Later that evening when Dan goes home, over a late dinner he has some surface talk about the day-to-day activities of the house. During the conversation, if there is a disagreement, Susan, as usual, concedes the point with a squashed sense of defeat. Dan, for once, senses this. The dialogue is not easy, and the air is strained. It's like they're both walking on eggshells around each other in their own ways. After his conversation with Cindy today, Dan is unwillingly in touch with just how bad things are between him and Susan. But what he sees is only the tip of the iceberg, because their problems go much deeper than he suspects or understands.

Dan tries to broach the issue of the tension in their relationship in an indirect way, but Susan quickly turns to mundane topics to keep the conversation on the surface. After trying to bring the conversation back to his topic of concern two or three times, Dan finally gets the message that Susan just doesn't want to talk about it. Dan is his own worst critic. He knows what a hard-ass he is on everyone, especially Susan and Carol, but he just can't help himself. He knows how he has alienated them and driven them away with his constant criticism and judgmentalism. Dan mentions the dive workshop as an indirect way of acknowledging that he knows he needs to change. Susan is distant and uninterested in discussing it any further. It is like she has crossed some inner line, and has just stopped caring either way.

After Susan heads to bed, Dan has a deep sense that something has to change. Maybe the dive workshop is the answer he needs at this point in time. Dan looks at the Web site for the dive workshop and downloads the information. To his surprise, he starts to get excited about the diving and the possibility of real change, and decides to book the trip. The next morning at breakfast, Dan chatters on about the dive workshop and flashes amazing pictures of underwater sea life that he downloaded and printed from the Web site the night before. He tries to explain to Susan that the workshop is about more than just scuba diving, that it teaches the principles of deep, profound, sustainable personal change. Susan sees an excitement in Dan that she hasn't seen in years. But all the same her expectations remain guarded.

Part of the requirement for enrollment was that each attendee had to complete an extensive self-scoring personality profile called the Riso-Hudson Enneagram Type Indicator (RHETI).[2] A copy of the RHETI was sent with the registration package that Dan received. After completing the questions, Dan scored as an Enneagram Type One. Type Ones are principled, orderly, self-controlled, perfectionistic, and self-righteous. "They are teachers, crusaders, and advocates for change: always striving to improve things, but afraid to make a mistake."[3]

Workshop attendees also had to complete a 360-degree review that was penetrating in scope and included asking a specified group of people (in Dan's case: Susan, Carol, Cindy, a couple of friends, and a few work colleagues) to evaluate them and send the results (which they would not reveal to Dan) back to the workshop instructor. Susan and Carol were shocked when they received the questions from the 360-degree review asking for detailed feedback on Dan. They knew that if they were really honest, they would burn a lot of bridges with him, but these were desperate times and honest feedback was the only kind they were willing to provide. Dan filled out his portion of the material, sent it back, then quickly forgot about anything to do with the dive workshop as he became once again caught up in the pressure of everyday life. Then, suddenly, the day of departure arrived.

THE ANTICIPATION OF ADVENTURE

There's nothing but deep, blue ocean between L.A. and Taipei—absolutely nothing. Dan settles into his business class seat on Singapore Airlines after a tight connection on his flight from JFK. Like every diver who heads off on a trip that takes him halfway around the world, Dan hopes the dive gear he checked in with his luggage is sitting beneath him somewhere in the cargo space of his plane, not back on some loading dock at LAX.

Dan has traveled extensively in the U.S. and Europe—so much so that he is flying free on airline miles. But he has never been to Asia. He is on his way to places he has only heard about. He does not have a visual picture of which country is next to which. Where is Vietnam relative to Laos and Malaysia, and where are these countries in relation to his destination, Bali, an island in Indonesia? Dan pulls the flight magazine from the seat pocket as the plane levels off at a cruising altitude of thirty-five thousand feet. He flips to the map at the back hoping to get some visual sense of where exactly he is going on this twenty-four thousand mile trip. His itinerary is New York to Los Angeles, L.A. to Taipei, Taipei to Singapore, and then on to Denpasar, the capital city of Bali.

The archipelago nation of Indonesia spans a three thousand mile arc from the mainland of Southeast Asia to Papua, New Guinea. Composed of almost eighteen thousand islands, only one thousand of which are inhabited, Indonesia covers about two million square miles of tropical seas, with over sixty thousand miles of coastlines, and is home to 15 percent of all the coral reefs in the entire world. Scientists believe that Indonesia is the place where all sea life originated. The density and diversity of life there is almost overwhelming, having twice the species of fish, coral, and invertebrates as the Great Barrier Reef of Australia. With every five hundred to a thousand miles that you move away from

Indonesia, you lose five hundred to a thousand species of marine organisms.

Indonesia is one of the largest nations in the world with over 210 million inhabitants, most of whom are Muslims. Nestled in the western part of Indonesia is Bali, the island of the gods, where the population is about 95 percent Balinese Hindu. Bali is densely populated in the eastern portion of the island, having over three million people total in an area of about 350 square miles.

Dan looks at the size of the Atlantic, then back to the Pacific, and has a new understanding of why people call flying to Europe "a hop across the pond." The visual image of the Pacific Ocean and the distance of just the first two flight segments forces the reality on him that he is going a long, long way from his home in Westchester County, New York.

After a fitful night of sleep on the fourteen-hour flight from L.A. to Taipei, and nodding in and out of consciousness on the segments to Singapore and then on to Bali, Dan has crossed the dateline and lands in Denpasar three calendar days after leaving New York. When he walks off the plane in Bali, he is confronted with a sensual overload of sights, smells, and sounds. The airport itself is a cultural experience, with people pressing him from all directions to buy things, change money, carry his bags, or get a taxi into town. Dan shakes these people off and walks to the luggage carousel, to wait for his luggage and dive gear with an air of inner pressure and tension from the chaos around him.

Dan is nervous enough that he hasn't dove in three years, but if the airline has lost his gear and he has to get unfamiliar rental gear, that will be just one more pressure and unfamiliarity. For Dan, the first few dives are always stressful, but once he gets back into the hang of it, he can begin to relax and enjoy the underwater world. He's relieved when he finally spots his dive gear bag amidst the other hundred dive gear bags, all of which are black.

As he clears customs, Dan walks out into the main airport terminal that is every bit as frenetic as Grand Central Station, but in very different ways. There must be thirty drivers holding signs with people's names on them and a crowd of young Balinese men yelling, "Taxi, taxi mister, please." Others are clamoring to help him with his luggage in the hopes of getting a tip. They are trying to eke out an existence in a country where two hundred U.S. dollars per month is considered a respectable salary. Dan never lets these people help him with his luggage. He always carries his own. He likes to be in control, especially in a place where he feels things could get out of hand very easily. A few young men press him to carry his luggage as he looks impatiently for a person holding a sign that has his name on it, and continually says, "No, no thank you," to people who couldn't seem to take no for an answer. In the short time he's been there, he's already annoyed to the point of anger. He brushes them aside as he pushes his way through the crowd without making any eye contact. Dan's view was that dealing with pressing crowds of people was like dealing with dogs—the first rule was never make eye contact.

Dan finally spots his name on a sign and recognizes the logo for the dive workshop. He's the last of four workshop participants who will be on this bus, so the driver says, "Okay, you have everything? Let's go to the bus." In the confusion of people pressing in on him one of the young men takes Dan's bags and says in broken English, "I carry to the bus." Dan somehow thinks he is with the dive workshop so he agrees. By the time they get outside, Dan notices that all the other people were carrying their own gear, and he instantly knows what has happened. He feels tricked, but knows he will have the last say. He lets the young man load all of his gear on the bus in the sweltering heat and then turns to get on the bus.

"Something for me?" the young man asks.

Dan, playing dumb, says, "What?" as if he does not understand.

Trying to speak in his very best English the man repeats, "Something for me, sir?"

"I don't know what you mean," is Wright's reply as he moves closer to the steps that lead onto the bus.

"A tip for me?" the young man pleads.

Dan halfway looks at him and says, "I have no money for a tip," and walks up the steps of the bus knowing that the young man is powerless against this rich American tourist who is part of a local tour. The Balinese man who is driving the bus sees it all, and in disgust shrugs his shoulders in sympathy for the young man. As the bus pulls away, the young man is angry and shocked at Dan's hardness of heart. Sticking to his rule, Dan never makes eye contact.

Dan sits next to a tall man named James. Dan asks James where he's from and ventures other pieces of small talk. But James gives him short perfunctory answers to his questions and that is the end of the conversation as far as James is concerned. James's style creates a kind of psychological space around him that says, "Leave me alone." This actually unnerves and annoys Dan, who is always friendly, but he gets the message and says no more to James.

Before the bus can fully stop at one intersection, ten to fifteen skinny boys descend upon it, brandishing newspapers and plastering them up against the side windows where the passengers were sitting. From across the aisle, Lindsey Barker starts commenting to Dan about the guys pressing the papers against the windows. The driver then volunteers that he had bought a paper in English the other day, and it wasn't until the light turned and he had driven away that he realized the paper was a week old.

~~~~~

Lindsey's chubby build, short brown hair, and wire-rimmed glasses gave her a matronly look of every person's mother. Relationships and helping others had always been the single most important thing in Lindsey's life. If you were to ask her, she would go on and on about how much she adored her mom and dad. But somehow she came away from her childhood feeling like she was not allowed to have her own needs in life, and this vacuum created an insatiable drive to be needed by others. She never felt wanted just for herself, but only when she was doing things for others. Service was the road to being loved and feeling close to people both inside and outside her home. Lindsey took the Enneagram a few years ago as part of a workshop on personal change, and it wasn't a surprise to her when she scored as an Enneagram Type Two this time on the RHETI. Type Twos are caring, interpersonal people who are empathetic, sincere, and warm-hearted. "They are friendly, generous, and self-sacrificing, but can also be sentimental, flattering, and people-pleasing."[4]

Lindsey was the Human Resources (HR) Director at a Long Island company that did primarily defense-related work. During the Clinton years, the company went through numerous and devastating downsizing exercises as they lost one government contract after another. But after September 11, 2001, the tap of defense revenues had once again begun to flow from Washington to the island, and Lindsey had been under the gun to increase the company's staff by 30 percent almost overnight. Not only did she succeed at this superhuman task, but she was able to snatch up some of the most qualified people on Long Island because of her personal connections and how quickly she moved.

The president of the company, Mario, had come to view her as an indispensable part of the management team. Mario was primarily a technical person who had few if any interpersonal skills either in the office or at home. He relied heavily on Lindsey to balance him out and he had come to trust her to handle the human side of the equation for the company, as well as making suggestions on sending his wife flowers when he forgot their anniversary. Over the years, Lindsey had become the informal power behind the throne and everyone knew that going up against her in a meeting or on a major decision was like committing organizational suicide. While she always did it in private, she was the only person in the company who could put Mario in his place.

What the senior staff saw that Lindsey and Mario didn't was her thinly disguised inner conflict between wanting to be a loyal resource for Mario, and wanting to run the company from behind the scenes. Her incessant comments about how brilliant Mario was and what great insight he had in his handling of the *technical* side of the house, left them with an inference that she was running the *administrative* side of the house, including their departments. In meetings, this gave other staff members the sickening feeling of out-and-out flattery, sometimes to the point of brownnosing. Mario didn't seem to object—he probably even enjoyed it.

Lindsey radiated a thinly veiled and inflated sense of pride in her own importance. She gave to get. Even her insistence that Mario allow her to organize the annual staff awards dinner to recognize high-performers in the company seemed to some to be simply a way for her to call attention to herself.

Her family and friends knew her to be compassionate and loving, a person who did not hold back her affection and was always ready to give people a big hug when they were down about something. Lindsey listened well if friends or family were hurting and she always seemed to know how to empathize and support them in a non-judgmental way. But those closest to Lindsey were as aware of some of the same blind spots as her colleagues were. She would constantly tell her friends and family how she really wanted to "be there" for them, but when push came to shove, she was noticeably absent when they needed her most.

She was overly aware of her positive and supportive feelings about them, but Lindsey had another, darker side to her that she seemed to have little or no consciousness of. What those closest to her found most destructive was that every *overt* thing that Lindsey did for them seemed to have a *covert* price of guilt and manipulation attached to it. When they backed away from this type of interaction, Lindsey would redouble her efforts to do more and try to get closer to them. Lindsey was a strange paradox of giving more than any person you knew, but at the same time coming across more emotionally needy than any person you knew. On the rare occasions when someone would confront her about her dark side, she would respond that she was just trying her best to care for them and be there for them. They were confused about why this type of "caring" left them feeling like they had just been punched in the stomach.

In addition to the support she provided to Mario and managing the ten-person Human Resources Office, Lindsey taught workshops in coaching skills, personal effectiveness, time management, and conflict resolution, as well as actually facilitating meetings and situations where there was enormous interpersonal conflict. Lindsey was on the board of directors of the Society of Human Resource Managers, and had made numerous presentations on HR-related areas, in which she was considered a nationally recognized expert on conflict management and personal effectiveness.

Lindsey had repeatedly told Mario that she was concerned about the demographics of the company because 60 percent of all employees were in the second half of life. She had been pressing Mario to develop a comprehensive staffing and career development plan. This was a process she would design and lead if Mario were to just give her the go-ahead.

Lindsey had learned to dive in the chilly waters off Long Island, but joined a scuba diving club so she could make periodic dive trips to the warm, clear waters of the Caribbean. She found out about the dive workshop through a friend who had attended and recommended it to her. Outwardly, she said she was going to the workshop to look for practical tools to take back to the office and help her gain new insights for her personal effectiveness workshop, as well as developing her plan for dealing with the aging staff at the company. But inwardly, she had a deeper connection to the aging staff than she was even aware of. She too was approaching the second half of life and had been feeling an increasingly powerful imperative to live her life to the fullest, rather than always living her life for others.

Lindsey had seen glimpses of her power-driven dark side in meetings and in interactions with family and friends. But she could not yet fully allow this hidden part of her into consciousness because it was so contradictory to everything she stood for. Lindsey honestly wanted to know her deeper self better, and to walk the road less traveled, but she didn't know where to find this inner road.

From behind the seat Dan is sitting in, Maggie Spinner is also making small talk with Dan and Lindsey, commenting on the five-story Hindu statues that were the focal point of the circle at every major intersection. Maggie says that she is from Colorado, and after filling her in on where he lives, Dan migrates into a discussion about how much he used to like to ski in Colorado. Lindsey chimes in saying that she's a skier too. James is also from Colorado, but true to form, he makes no attempt to join in on the conversation.

RELAXING AROUND THE POOL AT THE SWASTIKA

Thirty minutes later they arrive at the Swastika Hotel in Sanur, Bali, where they will be able to relax all day, do some local sightseeing, and leave for the boat bright and early tomorrow. The swastika is an ancient Balinese Hindu symbol that is a visual image of the rotation of the sun across the sky. Hitler borrowed it for the symbol of the German Third Reich. Of all the thousands of temples in Bali, nine of them are called directional temples because they are built in locations around the island so as to represent the north, south, east, and west points of this little island in relation to the celestial motion of the sun and planets. Every family compound and every other temple is oriented around these nine directional temples. In Bali, a person's position in the social structure is defined by the three-level caste system, and the anchoring of the heavenly world to the land of rice paddies with the nine directional temples defines every Balinese person's position in the cosmos.

The Swastika Hotel is laid out like a traditional Balinese family compound where rooms are like individual little huts, each with its own covered area to relax. In the center of the compound are two inviting pools set in the midst of lush gardens with the faint fragrance of exotic flowers and the sounds of birds that Dan has not heard before. When he arrives at the pool, he sees Maggie relaxing under a palm tree, drinking a cold beer, and looking over a book on diving in Indonesia. Maggie, a short, muscular blonde, who is forty but can pass for twenty-five, looks like she has been poured into her one-piece bathing suit. Dan sits down to chat and they talk about dive gear, the trip, where they are from, what they do, and how they have come to be on the trip.

Dan goes to get them both another beer at the pool bar, and as he looks back at Maggie sitting by the pool, he just can't take his eyes off her smooth, inviting body. Dan always had to manage his desire for other women. Maggie reminded him of the time when he met Cheryl, a sales rep for an electronics supplier. They had had drinks, one thing led to another and soon Cheryl had her hand on Dan's leg under the table. He told her she had to stop, but he really didn't want her to and she knew that. They went for dinner, walked to Cheryl's SUV, and made love to each other in the back of the truck far into the night. This totally contradicted everything Dan stood for, and while he had loved every minute of it, he snapped his stoic self-control back into place, called Cheryl the next day and told her it was a mistake, and that it could never happen again. From then on, Dan would have flirtatious liaisons with women who allowed him to get close, but not too close. He justified this in his mind by saying that he could look, briefly touch, but not go all the way. In reality, these so-called friendships were a way for him to play out his sexual fantasies, while staying within the outer bounds of his legalistic rules of self-conduct.

Maggie had always been the quintessential image of success, who had hammered her way to the top of every challenge she had taken on by the power of her raw, unmitigated, competitive will. She had heard about the Enneagram through her studies, but knew little about it until she scored as an Enneagram Type Three and began reading the description of her type. Type Threes are adaptable, success-oriented people who are self-assured, attractive, and charming. They are "ambitious, competent, and energetic, they can also be status-conscious and highly driven for advancement."[5]

Maggie grew up on a farm in the Midwest, and for as long as she could remember she never felt that it was okay for her to have her own feelings, or her own identity as a person. She didn't feel loved for who she was, independent of her achievements, successes, and superhuman victories in life. In her mind, the ticket to feeling valued by people was to succeed—which only increased her drive to continue succeeding. Her life was a fast-moving treadmill, and at forty she was really, really tired of forever running the race of life.

Maggie was Vice President of Public Relations for a large chemical corporation near Rocky Flats, Colorado. She lived in the cultural center of Boulder and had been doing graduate level studies in spirituality and world religions at CU Boulder for some time now. Maggie's twenty-year-old daughter, Rena, was the only reminder of a long-gone marriage that Maggie never talked about out of a deep sense of shame. Rena attended Colorado College, a small, private, liberal arts school in Colorado Springs, and on weekends and over school breaks she and Maggie would spend time skiing, hiking, biking, and scuba diving, which Maggie had learned years earlier.

Maggie and Rena were riding up the chair lift to the bowl high above the Winter Park ski area and Maggie started chatting with Troy, one of the ski instructors. It was his day off and he offered to show them around the mountain, so Maggie and Rena got the royal tour of the best skiing that Winter Park had to offer, followed by cocktails in the hot tub at the townhome complex where Troy lived. Maggie was used to being treated like royalty. She was stunningly beautiful in a healthy, outdoor-looking way, and her firm, sexually alluring body almost always turned men's heads. Many a guy who competed for the "privilege" of waiting on her hand and foot called her a queen, but only on his way out of the door of her life. More than anything, men and women had accused her of being vain, but since she had all the goods to back her image up, she just dismissed this commentary as the envy of those who were the ugly people in life.

Troy had studied philosophy at CU Boulder, and since the only thing his degree enabled him to do was to go to graduate school, he decided to take a job as a ski instructor and see if any new direction came into his life. That was fifteen years ago, and Troy hadn't looked back since. Troy was a different kind of guy—introspective, connected to the deeper things in life, sensitive to people, and intent on finding a sense of meaning and contribution in life. He was an incredibly good-looking guy who had done some modeling for ski magazines, but unlike Maggie, he wasn't pretentious about it—he just was what he was.

Over the next year, Maggie spent more time at Troy's place in Winter Park than she did at her house in Boulder and she found herself falling in love with Troy in a way that she had never experienced before. In the summer, they would go for hikes in the mountains and Maggie would feel an inner sense of freedom as she let her feet dangle in the crystal clear, cold water of a Colorado mountain stream. As winter came they would trek into the backcountry on snowshoes and overnight in backcountry huts that overlooked the continental divide. Troy was not like the other men that she had been with and somehow he was waking up emotions and a vision for her life that she had never felt before. But what she found most interesting was that Troy was completely unimpressed with her image and the emphasis that she put on competing about almost everything and being the best at any price.

At the office, Maggie had been thrust into the middle of an enormous corporate crisis and she was at the focal point of the action. Local environmental groups had become more and more insistent and vocal that her company was secretly dumping chemicals into the ground upstream of their city's aquifer. As the Vice President of Public Relations, she was forced to face off with these people, who hounded her night and day and had even begun calling her at home. Maggie was able to counteract every allegation with a masterful combination of factual information, spin control, and, when necessary, smoke and mirrors. Every attack they mounted, she was able to disarm. She tried to give the impression that she really cared for them and their concerns, but under these thinly veiled lies she disdained this bunch of environmental do-gooders and whiners. The company president, J.R., and the Board of Directors were pleased and relieved that Maggie seemed to be winning this war of words, factoids, and emotions that played out daily on the front pages of the Denver Post.

But during her field research to refute one of the environmental-ist's claims, Maggie discovered an underground discharge pipe from the plant that was not on any of the facility drawings. When she began to inquire about it, no one in the company seemed to know about it. Then she found herself summoned to J.R.'s office where she was emphatical-ly instructed to stop asking questions about the discharge pipe and to just stick to the fine job she had been doing defeating those people's claims. But as she secretly did more field research, she became increas-ingly convinced that the company was indeed discharging poisonous chemicals underground and that the local environmental groups were right in their allegations.

Maggie had a tendency to put her psychological energy into being what people wanted to see, making a good impression, form over sub-stance, and coming across well. Troy saw a different side of Maggie, deep below the surface of her charm, white lies, and cool-and-calculat-ed image. Despite her singular focus on success, Troy saw in her the power to be inner-directed, to be driven by the value of helping others, regardless of whether or not it led to success. Certainly she was ambi-tious, but her best side was when she used this drive to grow psychologically and improve herself. Troy wasn't sure that *Maggie* could see this deeper part of herself that was committed to integrity, because she had locked it away in a compartment somewhere deep in her per-sonality. On the occasions when it pounded its way to freedom and escaped, she tended to rationalize and disown this part of her true self so she could keep up the show and go on performing.

Maggie had left the office for the weekend troubled in a way that she'd never been troubled before. The drive into the snow-covered foothills to the west of Boulder, up over the eleven thousand-foot pass and down into the secluded valley where Winter Park sits, was a time of quiet reflection and soul searching for Maggie. One of the things she always looked forward to was to sit in the hot tub with Troy looking toward the runs of the ski area and just talk about their day, their week, and what they wanted from each other and life. That day, she poured her heart out to Troy about the discharge pipe she had discovered. He was really taken aback, but not totally surprised because he never really trusted J.R.

Troy said, "Why don't you just put the evidence you have in an envelope to the reporter at the Denver Post who has been covering the story, then walk into J.R.'s office and just quit?"

"I can't do that," Maggie protested.

"Why not?" Troy pressed. "I'll bet you could make decent money tending bar here at night in the base lodge, ski all day, and not have to burden yourself with these corporate problems and the pressure to lie and cover up just to keep your job."

Monday morning, she was back on the job defending the company and defeating the arguments of the local environmentalists, but now she was doing her job knowing that they were right.

Maggie was trying to decide if she should take Troy's advice, and she had use-or-lose vacation time building up, so she decided to attend the dive workshop, and put off the decision about confronting J.R. until after she got back. She knew she was good at what she did—in fact, she was probably the best in the business. But when she was honest with herself, and looked inside and asked who she was independent of her professional image, she had no idea. That scared her to the depths of her soul. Troy saw things in her that she did not, and their relationship had mirrored those things so powerfully that she was finally starting to get a glimmer of them for herself. Maggie was tiring of the image and persona she had worn all her life. She was hungering for some integrity. She had a hounding thirst for authenticity. She wanted to be real for the first time in her life, but she didn't know exactly how to go about satisfying these deep needs and desires. Troy could have come to the dive workshop, but Maggie felt that she needed the psychological space to explore her inner confusion alone.

~~~~~

It is almost 3:00 P.M. and the sun is scalding Dan and Maggie to the point where even the cold beer and the pool can barely keep them comfortable. Maggie begins picking up her things to leave, and says, "Well, I think I'm going to head up to my room and cool off." Dan wishes he was going with her, and without thinking says, "How about having dinner together tonight?" After a slight pause she says, "Sure, what time?"

They meet at the restaurant next door at 7:00 P.M. Dinner is a mixture of eating Indonesian food and exchanging stories about diving, business, travel, and relationships. Dan is quite taken with Maggie. She's bright, energetic, and full of a sense of adventure about the trip and even about the choices she is facing in life. Dan charges the meal to his room and says, "Why don't we wander back to the hotel?"

When they reach the front desk of the hotel to get their room keys, Maggie abruptly says, "Well, I'm going to call it a night. I'll see you in the morning." Dan is disappointed, but hides it. "Sure, see ya tomorrow."

~~~~~

Most of the dive workshop participants are staying at the Swastika and they meet in the lobby at 7:30 A.M. for the twenty-five-minute bus ride to Benoa harbor, where they will board the ship,

Explorer. The *Explorer* is a traditional Balinese sailing ship that is powered by a 454-horsepower diesel engine, but can also run with the wind under the power of two enormous main sails and a jib. When they pull up to the dock and are able to see all 110 feet of her length and the thirty-two feet of her beam, the reality of what they are about to embark upon begins to sink into their heads. The workshop leader, Thomas Rose, greets them as they board the boat. With light brown curly hair around the sides of his balding head, Thomas has deep blue searching eyes and is about twenty-five pounds overweight. After some chitchat about peoples' trips, and initial impressions about the boat, Thomas says that he wants to set sail as soon as possible. Various crewmembers then show Dan and the others to their cabins.

Dan is in Cabin 2 in the front of the boat and had requested the lower bunk because he frequently has to go to the bathroom in the middle of the night. The cabin door swings open with a bang, and in walks James, the quiet guy from the bus. James and Dan will be roommates over the next six days and neither one is all that thrilled about that prospect. Despite the fact that James wanted the bottom bunk, he says his perfunctory "Hi" then proceeds to unpack his gear.

James Tuffs, a six-foot-six, brown-eyed, olive skinned bodybuilder whose enormously developed chest and arms show through even the loosest shirts, had always pushed people's boundaries. Although his parents never came right out and said it to him, their cold and distant relationship gave him the clear message that he was on his own in life. Even in his teen years, James honestly believed that given the right circumstances anyone, even his closest friend or a family member would screw him over. James trusted no one. He rarely let people get too close to him, and when he didn't really know someone, he sent out the loud message that they should just *stay away*. He also got very uncomfortable about giving out too much information about himself to people he didn't know well. When James read the description of his Enneagram Type Eight, he found that it nailed him dead on. Type Eights are powerful and aggressive people who are self-confident, strong and assertive. They are "protective, resourceful, straight-talking, and decisive, but can also be ego-centric and domineering."[6]

James got his undergraduate degree in structural engineering from Texas A&M and then decided to go on to law school in Austin. Before he even graduated, he was recruited by a well-established law firm in Dallas and within five years he was told that they were considering making him a partner. James's case load focused primarily on high-stakes, high dollar divorce and custody cases where he quickly earned the reputation of being a hired gun—a verbally abusive, in-your-face kind of guy who could get his clients the blacktop off the opponent's driveway if they wanted it.

James always made sure that he dominated the people in his professional life, and even used his power and strength to control the direction of his personal relationships. If James was not in the power position, he was uncomfortable with himself, and the life he had was hammered into existence by the sheer force of his will.

Paul Henderson, the senior partner who had recruited James and had told him about the firm's intention to make him a partner, found a summer job for his eighteen-year-old daughter Tonya as a paralegal. When Tonya started flirting with James, he pounced on her sexually with an insatiable lust that was more like power than love. They were together as much as possible. Tonya even convinced James to take her to the Cayman Islands for a week where they both got certified to scuba dive. Tonya loved the attention and the unbridled sex, that is, until she got pregnant toward the end of the summer. With the school year approaching quickly, Tonya got an abortion, which was just fine with James, who didn't want that kind of responsibility. Tonya demanded that James stay away from her, but James rarely capitulated to demands of any kind. Three weeks later, Tonya left for school, which she hoped would solve her "James problem" and let her move on with her life.

Two years had passed since James had been told about the prospect of becoming a partner in the firm, but there was no sign of any movement in this direction. James had asked around about it a few times, and finally was able to pry the secret loose that Paul had lobbied the other senior partners not to extend the offer to James as payback for what had happened with his daughter, Tonya. Regardless, James felt he had been betrayed. With full-on vengeance, he turned his verbally abusive, in-your-face attitude on Paul in meetings within the firm and even in front of clients. Weeks of this turned into months, and the tension in the firm was so thick you could cut it with the proverbial knife. Other senior partners began challenging James on his behavior and attitude toward Paul. But James refused to back down—they'd promised him a partnership and then reneged because of something that was totally unrelated to his performance. When some of their largest and longest-standing clients began to complain to Paul and the other senior partners about James, the partners decided they had to begin the process of building a file of objective evidence against James, then show him to the door.

James had developed a tightly woven and small group of friends and confidants in Dallas who he allowed to see below the turbulent, often violent, surface of his life. They knew him to be a natural-born leader who people wanted to follow, and an honorable person who would use his strength, control, and power to help them and even protect them if necessary. Once you were in the inner circle, James would go against all odds to make sure the world did not take advantage of or harm you.

But once you betrayed James, there was no going back, and James made it very difficult not to cross him at some point in time. People who had betrayed him described him as a loose cannon who went off without warning, a guy who would fight at the drop of a hat and wore it tipped to start with, like he had some hidden score to settle with life. James kept an unbridgeable psychological moat between him and people outside the inner circle because he figured the less they knew about him, the less they could use against him.

One night during a family dinner over winter break, Tonya heard her father, Paul, complaining about James and the plans they had to fire him. Tonya suspected what the problem was, but the topic was "off limits" with her father. All Tonya had to do was let things run their course, and her problem with James would be over for good. Within weeks of her return to school, the senior partners unanimously voted to remove James from the firm, buying him off with an overly liberal separation package effective immediately. The speed of their action took James by surprise, and after trying to sabotage as many client relationships as he could, he turned his caseload over to the others in the firm, and stormed out of the building, knocking over anything within his reach. Paul was just glad to be rid of him.

James wiped the dust off his feet and got a real change of lifestyle by moving to Alma, Colorado, a place he had been camping near for the last few summers. Alma is a town of two hundred people. It is two blocks wide, four blocks long and, at an elevation of 10,587 feet above sea level, it is the highest town in North America. Alma is pure, ungentrified Colorado, only fifteen miles south of the world-class ski resort at Breckenridge. When James got to Alma, he rented a small house about a mile off the road that ran through town. It was quiet there—so quiet that the only thing James heard when he sat on his front porch in the evening was the thunderous sound of his own breath. He picked up a copy of the *Fairplay Flume* in the post office where he had to go to get his mail, and scoured the half page of want ads looking for a job. He wanted to do anything but be a lawyer. With his background in engineering, he easily landed a job as one of Park County's two building inspectors.

James had his share of trouble as an inspector. Park County was like a different universe from the world he had just left. Nobody cared who he was, what he knew, or where he went to law school. In Alma, how much you knew was more closely tied to how long you'd been in town and whether you remembered Alma when Main Street was still a dirt road. James was no respecter of persons in a rural setting that was all about nepotism, old friendships and how many generations people had been ranching in Park County. One day over a beer at the South Park Saloon, his neighbor, Bobby, told James that he had been living in Alma for twenty-five years, and the old-timers still did not consider him a "local." Whether he was dealing with contractors, county commissioners, long-time locals, or his small group of new friends, James tried to dominate them and force his opinions and views on them. He would push, and push, and push some more until he had totally alienated people. Occasionally, someone who cared about him even less than he cared about them would push him back with equally abusive, intimidating, and street-wise force. James accepted this for what it was. He always respected a worthy adversary on the few occasions that he found one.

Ten years of the quiet, solitary, reflective life in the high country began to change James. Over the years, he flirted with the idea of opening a law office, but was increasingly taunted by remorse and inner conflict about the families he had helped to tear apart in the courtroom. He was also taunted by how abusive and vengeful he had been to people, but he had been that way for as long as he could remember. He had little prospect for real change. James had left a broad, long trail of psychological damage and shameful situations behind him. In the quietness and peace of the mountains, when the normal distractions of life were not there to drown them out, the inner voices of shame and remorse haunted him and became harder and harder to push to the fringe of his consciousness.

Despite surface appearances, James had always been a deeply spiritual person. Although he had little use for religion, he began attending the small Episcopal Church in Breckenridge, because the Episcopalians were the only group of Christians who were liberal and open enough to accept him for who he was. James took comfort in the fact that normally the sermon was slightly over twelve minutes, so he didn't have to sit through the typical judgmental diatribe that most preachers dispensed, the kind of moralizing that kept him out of church for most of his life. The way the liturgy was set up, they always said the Nicene creed after the sermon, so even if the priest was preaching heresy, James always got a little grounding in the truth anyway.

Victoria was a successful technical writer who lived and worked in Denver and who owned a condo on Peak Eight in Breckenridge. Victoria was staying at her condo for the weekend, and she and James met and talked during the coffee time following the service, then James asked her if she had plans for lunch. Within eighteen months, James and Victoria were married and had their first child on the way. They bought a piece of land just two miles north of Alma and designed and built a log home high above the floor of Placer Valley. Victoria always called it a log *home*, never a *house,* because what she and James were building went beyond a structure to live in, it was a home in the truest sense James had ever known. He would always get a kick out of telling his friends back in the flat, hot, humid, dusty plains around Dallas that he was living at over eleven thousand feet at eye level with snow-covered peaks and eagles, just north of a town of two hundred people.

Victoria was the first woman that James had ever really loved, because she was the only woman who was strong enough to put him in his place when he needed to be. More than anyone else, Victoria saw beneath James' hardened and calcified exterior and she loved him as no one had ever loved him. James may have been tough, but he was no fool—he saw this quality in Victoria and he honored it and honored her as his wife.

But even more than Victoria, it was Jon and Julia, their two children, who reached into the depths of a heart that had been hardened by decades of conflict, interpersonal war, and vengeance. Friends who were close to James had told him that more than anything else, it was the birth of his children that had changed him from the hard recalcitrant self that he fostered for most of his life. James's instincts told him that there was something to this, but he wasn't exactly sure how children, who he had refused to have for so many years because of the responsibility they involved, could in the second half of his life have such a deep and abiding effect upon him. For the first time, James was a part of a family who actually cared for him, and this experience of warmth and intimacy was comforting and at the same time terrifying. Intimacy was what he defended against all his life, but intimacy turned out to be exactly what he had needed.

Building inspectors don't make much, and inspectors in Park County make even less, so James decided to open a law office on Main Street in Alma, next to Alma's Only Bar. During the days that led to his opening the office, James fought with the demons of his soul that taunted him and intensified his guilt and remorse about the families he had helped to destroy as an attorney and the way he'd lived his life. In some strange way, the comfort of his own family sometimes intensified the damage he had done to the lives of others. But James approached this new practice from a different perspective, one of helping people who could not help themselves, and might become the victims of hateful, manipulating lawyers like he used to be. He knew intuitively that this was the right path, but he had no idea where this path would lead him. James quickly gained a reputation as the best lawyer in the north part of Park County, which was rural and mountainous, but geographically as large as the state of Rhode Island. Within two years, his practice grew to the point where he had to hire a full-time paralegal to help him.

Despite the financial success of his practice, James began to feel a strange inner stirring. When he was out walking his dog or hiking in the solitude of Mt. Bross high above his home, and stopped long enough to connect to his deep feelings, they seemed like an emotional "wound" in the depths of his soul. James felt a deep inner restlessness about what he was doing and where he was going in life. His law practice made many things possible for his family that being a building inspector didn't, but he felt really tired of doing what he was doing. He found himself hungering for a deeper sense of meaning and contribution in his life, and he had no idea what would satisfy this hunger. He knew that he had embarked on some type of inner journey, but he had no idea where he was going, or how he was going to get there. James hadn't been diving for years, but signed up for the dive workshop hoping to find a new framework within which to understand what he was experiencing in his life. Victoria encouraged James to go to the dive workshop because she had seen how the inner pressure for change was gnawing at him. More than anything, he hoped the dive workshop would help him find a clear path forward. He'd been to some of these kinds of workshops before and what worried him most was the prospect of having to endure too much touchy-feely stuff, joining hands around the proverbial campfire to sing songs, or any of that New Age metaphysical crap.

～～～～

Dan has finished unpacking his gear in the cabin and he and James exchange a few more perfunctory words, then Dan says, "I'll see you up on deck." As Dan climbs the stairs to the main deck he wonders how sharing a room with James will work out. Dan doesn't like room-mates any more than James appears to, so they are both going to have to make the best of it for the next six days.

Up on deck, people are unpacking their dive bags and putting their dive gear together. The crew is issuing homing beacons to each diver so if one of them is pulled out to sea by a strong current, they can be tracked from the boat. The device has the on-off switch taped down with duct tape because the crew said that switching it on activated an entire satellite network. Divers were only to remove the tape and acti-vate it when they were in an emergency situation. Just the fact that the crew issued this type of device puts the group on notice that they might be up against some challenging diving situations.

Thomas is setting up his dive gear, but at the same time he is looking around and watching the interaction between people and lis-tening to their conversations. Although the crew of the *Explorer* is responsible for leading the dives, Thomas's responsibility is to teach the dive workshop and to handle any negative interpersonal interactions that might occur. Thomas has been on enough live-aboard boats to know that at first people are always polite and get along, but after the first few days this veneer gets thin and the real personalities of the peo-ple start coming through. Then a kind of bifurcation sets in where people interact on two levels. They maintain the veneer of being pleas-ant, but underneath it all people really start to get on one another's nerves. Thomas is the kind of person who picks up on this even when he doesn't care to. He is like a radio that's tuned to two stations simultaneously. While acting as if nothing's amiss, he can sense the dissonance between people in their mannerisms, their tone of voice, and how they avoid each other. Normally this is as far as it goes, but occasionally the dissonance erupts and people actually get up in each other's faces. This doesn't happen often on live-aboard dive boats, but when it does, Thomas has to step in and break it up—quickly and decisively.

FOUNDATIONAL PRINCIPLES AND HOUSEKEEPING STUFF

The ship backs away from the dock and they begin the eighteen-hour sea journey to a small island off the coast of Sumbawa where they will dive tomorrow morning. Dan climbs to the upper deck to get a better view, grabs a deck chair and looks out over the vast blue sea that lies just outside the harbor—this is the ocean that he will soon be diving and exploring. A chill of excitement, tinged with trepidation, courses through his body.

There is an enormous cruise ship moored in the bay. Dan is fixated on it when someone standing near the wheelhouse says, "It's called the *Sea Journey*. It holds two thousand passengers plus one thousand crew and sails around the world." Dan is impressed. "Hi, my name is Kirsten," the person says. "I'm one of the dive instructors on the trip."

Kirsten is tall, slim, with blonde hair and bright blue eyes and has a slight European accent. She has been living in Bali for about six years, and had been diving up in Tulamben on the northwest coast where the diving was primarily "shore diving." Divers would simply step into the water from their resort and do a short surface swim of about one hundred feet offshore, where lurking beneath them, were some of the most magnificent coral reefs in the world. Originally from Sweden, Kirsten is a friendly and open person who fits right in with the Balinese locals, with whom she has made many lasting friendships. Last year, she moved to the south of Bali to join the crew of the *Explorer*.

Thomas rings the bell that signals an assembly and Dan excuses himself while Kirsten steps into the wheelhouse to say something to the captain. It is only 10:00 A.M. but it seems much later because they had gotten such an early start. One by one people begin coming from the different parts of the ship to take their places at the enormous wooden table in the center of the main deck. The table has a bright blue tarp overhead that protects people from the sun, yet allows the sea breeze to cool them even in the highest heat of the day. The table was designed as a space for underwater cameras and dive computers, but during this trip, it will serve as a teaching table around which the workshop will take place.

There are handouts, booklets, pens, and a logbook in front of each chair, and name tags for people to write their names on and stick to their shirts. Over toward the railing is a flip chart that is just barely under the blue tarp where Thomas is standing. This is the first time Dan has seen all of the other dive workshop participants face-to-face in one place. There are nine of them, including Thomas, and no one is below the age of thirty-five.

Thomas introduces Mike and Kirsten as the scuba instructors who will be leading the diving part of the workshop. "I will be doing all the dives with the group, so I'll just turn the floor over to them a little later on so they can give us the opening briefing on the boat and our dive procedure." With long, curly hair below his shoulders, Mike looks like a wild man. He has worked on dive boats in Palau, Fiji, and Papua New Guinea, among other places around the world. Originally from England, he is witty and bright, quick with his tongue—he has a kind of iconoclastic and cynical tone to everything he says. When Mike turns this cynical wit in your direction, you never know whether you should take him seriously and be upset that he is rude, or just laugh with him like it is all in good fun.

Standing at the flip chart on the main deck of the boat, Thomas speaks. "I want to begin with some opening remarks about the dive workshop material, and then Mike and Kirsten will give us an overview of the diving we are going to be doing. I want you to take the 3x5 card from your packet, get into an introspective space, and then jot down a few lines about what led you to come to the dive workshop and what you hope to get out of it. Don't put your name on the cards. When you're done, pass them up to me so I can read them over and get a better sense about the group's expectations for the next six days." A hush falls over the group as they focus on thinking and writing.

Rick Flowton didn't know what to write because he was there just to appease his father-in-law. Rick was medium height, thin, with black hair, almond-brown eyes that show his partly Asian background, and an awkward but friendly smile that was painted on his face. Rick had always been an easy-going guy who didn't like to make waves. He was raised in a family whose philosophy was that children should be seen, but not heard. He learned to scuba dive as a teenager, not because he wanted to, but because his family pressured him into it. Despite this, he came to like the sport. Whenever he tried to assert himself, people responded with a pressure for him to remain invisible—life just went on without him almost like his presence did not make a difference to the course of life. When Rick read the description of his Enneagram Type Nine, he thought some of it kinda sounded like him, but he wasn't really sure that it was a good description of how he was. Type Nines are easy-going, self-effacing people who are accepting, trusting, and stable. "They are usually creative, optimistic, and supportive, but can also be too willing to go along with others to keep the peace."[7]

Rick had lived with his wife Linda and three young children in a house he owned in Evanston, Illinois. He had gone to Northwestern, earned a degree in business, and had been the CFO of the Stonewall corporation, a small family-run business on the north side of Chicago. About six years ago, the originator of the company retired and gave control of the operation to his grandson Josh, who was bright and energetic and breathed new life and enthusiasm into a small business that had been maintaining the status quo for years. Josh's gung-ho approach paid off in bottom-line results as the company grew from $5 million per year to $80 million over a five-year period. Josh set his sights on managed growth that was driven by new marketing strategies, customer focus, and quantitative measures of employee performance to push productivity to the bottom-line.

Rick hated conflict more than anything and did everything he could to avoid it. His image of "the good life" was peace and harmony in all his relationships—a Norman Rockwell setting. But he never quite learned the lesson that when he put conflict off, it magnified, intensified, and only got worse. Time after time with professional, family, and friendship relationships, Rick would withdraw from facing difficulties whenever he could. In the end, putting conflict off forced him to deal with much more conflict than if he had just faced issues directly all along.

When Stonewall was first started, Rick was the lead man in a four person accounting office. Eight years later, Rick was promoted to CFO by Josh's grandfather and Rick's staff grew to over ten people. From the very beginning, Josh had serious questions about Rick's ability to handle the bigger operation, but his grandfather had confidence that Rick could grow with the company and should be given more and more responsibility. Rick was given assignments and performance targets, which he never completed on time. When Josh confronted him about his poor performance, Rick would insist that he was overworked and that he needed more staff. In the old days, this type of diversionary whining would work, and Rick would get more staff. But in the new performance-based culture that Josh was trying to establish, these cries fell on deaf ears. A desk audit that Josh asked the HR manager to conduct of Rick's actual day-to-day activities revealed that he was seriously under-employed. Casual, day-to-day observations of Rick showed that he spent more time gossiping with the "old timers" about how unhappy he was about the changes Josh was making in the company, and passive-aggressively undermining those changes at every turn. After discussing these issues with Rick informally on a number of occasions, Josh told the HR manager to begin documenting Rick's lack of performance on deliverables, as well as his duplicitous attempts to undermine the new organizational culture Josh was trying to bring to the company.

Rick was a strange mixture of a really nice guy who chatted with his employees over coffee in an approachable demeanor, and someone who had to maintain control by insisting that he be involved in every decision that was made in his department. Many of his people liked him, but a few hated him because they were always having to clean up the organizational messes that he left behind. His in-box was like a black hole, everything went in, nothing ever came out. Often quiet and unassuming in staff meetings, Rick was very subtly interested in his image, how big his office was, whether he got free parking privileges, and all the other trappings of organizational power. Out of loyalty to Rick, and a desire to see the company succeed, the staff who liked him worked around him and covered for him just to get the job done. The people who were terminally frustrated by his passive-aggressive undermining of Josh's new culture, and Rick's duplicitous support for Josh in meetings, would tell Josh what was really going on. Josh continued to build the paper file of Rick's poor performance. He tolerated Rick while his grandfather was still involved in the transition of the company, but once the responsibility for the company was fully his, firing Rick was the first high-level administrative decision that Josh would make.

Frank and Connie, Linda's parents, also had questions about Rick's level of motivation even before he got fired, lost his house, and moved Linda and the kids into their basement in the southwest suburbs of Chicago. Their moving in was only supposed to be until "things got straightened out," but Frank and Connie both had a bad feeling about how long this would take. Living with Rick and Linda allowed Frank to watch Rick's coming and going more closely, and he only made intermittent attempts to look for a job. It was a buyer's market for employers at that time where there were many more applicants than there were jobs. Most potential employers were able to see through the smoke screen of Rick's inflated history of titles, promotions, and "accomplishments." Others got the picture quickly when they called his former employer as a reference check. Rick even applied for government positions where he knew he could trade a reduction in his former salary for job security, but nothing turned up. Every rejection letter and unreturned phone call just drove Rick's self-esteem further into the ground. Beneath his nice guy exterior, Rick was depressed and felt like he was sinking into the muck and mire of the pressure and demands of a world that he just could not keep up with.

Rick would "check out" as a way of dealing with problematic situations or when the pressure of everyday life grew too intense. Unfortunately for the people in his life, when Rick didn't deal with his problems, *they* had to pick up the pieces as he just stood there with an unknowing, faraway stare in his eyes. Most people looked beyond his shortcomings because Rick was an open, easy-going person. In many ways, Rick actually had a kind of calming influence on difficult situations. But for those who were closest to him and saw him at his worst, he was an overly agreeable, too-submissive doormat who feared and resisted almost all change, regardless of the cost to himself or others.

Connie had been pushing Frank to do something to take the pressure off, but Frank was torn about getting involved. From the perspective of a CPA who owned an accounting firm, there was *no way* that Frank would give Rick a job working for him. But as a father who was concerned about the welfare of Linda and his grandchildren, he stewed over scenario after scenario of how he could help, without being one more enabler to Rick's indolence.

Frank had been observing a trend of how clients who lived up to thirty minutes north of his current location were traveling to use his services because there were no accounting firms in that immediate area. Connie was pushing Frank to open another location to the north, and to let Rick run that operation. They could rent office space, transfer some of the current staff and the more northern clients to that location, and let Rick build up the rest of the business. Given the fact that Rick was not a CPA, the northern branch would do bookkeeping, accounting, and taxes, and Frank would still do the CPA tasks. It sounded good on paper, but Frank was worried about the reality of it all.

Because Frank had chosen an excellent location in an area where there were no other accountants, and transferred three of his best staff and $175 thousand in existing client revenues to the new location, the business grew to about a quarter of a million dollars in a little over eighteen months. The growth was due primarily to the word of mouth marketing that happened because of the lead person on Rick's staff, Joanne. Joanne was an aggressive, competent go-getter who had worked for Frank for over ten years and handled some of the larger accounts that were transferred to the northern location. Clients who worked with Joanne liked her and told others, which served to make the business grow more rapidly. In fact, the growth happened in spite of Rick, who was back into the flow of the management style that had gotten him fired only two years earlier.

Joanne wanted to please Frank, but soon saw through the contradictions of Rick's management style. Rick would say yes, when he meant no. His words rarely matched his deeds. When Rick disagreed with Joanne, rather than confront the conflict, he would play dumb and say he didn't understand. Joanne learned quickly that when Rick said he didn't understand, what he was really saying was that he didn't agree. She was ready to strangle him because she hated the duplicity of his passive-aggressive style. As far as Joanne was concerned, passive-aggression was still aggression, and she spent a major portion of her time doing damage control with the other two people in the office who also saw through Rick. Joanne tried to broach the topic with Frank on numerous occasions, but this put both of them in the difficult position of sharing issues that were uncomfortable. As the conflict in the office grew, Rick predictably ignored it, hoping it would go away, and painted nothing but rosy pictures in his weekly reports to Frank, who knew better. Frank didn't want to rock the boat because Rick, Linda, and the children had finally moved out and into a new house and Frank didn't want them moving back in with them. So the real depth and magnitude of the problem was almost completely masked by the increase in clients and revenues and the only question was, when would Joanne just quit out of utter frustration.

About a year later, Joanne's non-compete agreement with the firm expired and Rick, who was responsible for renewing employee contracts, failed to notice this. Things had gone from bad to worse, and despite her continued discussions with Frank, nothing was being done and there was no change in sight. Joanne knew she was the backbone of the business because the clients she serviced were about 60 percent of the total revenues of the northern location, plus her reputation had brought in most of the new clients. She decided it was time for a show-down. She began confronting Rick on a regular basis in memos about his mismanagement of the business, with copies going to Frank. Rick would meet with her, admit that he needed to do better, but then noth-ing would change or he'd tell her he didn't completely understand what she wanted from him.

When Joanne could take it no more, she walked in, dropped her resignation on Frank's desk, and said, "I told you it was either Rick or me." Frank was speechless, and tried to smooth things over by taking her out for a farewell lunch to wish her well. Rather than rehash the problems about Rick yet one more time, they both decided to just chat about the good old days and things that were happening outside of the office. At one point close to the end of their meal, Frank asked Joanne what she planned to do next. Joanne replied that she was going to do some accounting work out of her house. Frank wished her well, having no idea what this would mean for him.

Within two weeks of Joanne's leaving, the majority of the big clients that she serviced had called Rick to tell him they were changing accountants. Although they didn't say why, it didn't take Frank long to figure out where the clients were going. Frank called and threatened Joanne with legal action, claiming she had a non-compete agreement that stated she could not run off with his clients. But the letter that Joanne's lawyer sent in response included a copy of the expired non-compete agreement, proving it had been out of force for almost a year, thus Frank had no legal recourse.

Frank grabbed the phone to discuss the factuality of the lawyer's letter with Rick. Rick said that the non-compete agreement was one of the things that had slipped through the cracks because he was so over-worked with the increase in clients and revenue, all of which he tried to take credit for. Rick had so many blind spots about what actually had gone on that he lashed out at Frank, claiming he was overworked and understaffed. So what was he supposed to do? Frank was incredulous at this round of lame excuses that only revealed how deeply Rick was unaware of his total lack of initiative, and his weak management style of pushing his own work off on others to the point where he had none.

Joanne's resignation had put Frank in a quandary. If he were to fire Rick for incompetence, as he rightly should, he would risk alienating his wife and daughter. They all knew that Rick would be unable to find another job with a similar salary. With a prolonged period of unemployment, Rick and Linda might lose their new house and have to move back in with Frank and Connie. But if he kept Rick, how could he salvage the northern location with the weight of Rick's incompetence around his neck? Like Joanne had told him so many times before, Frank would have to continue to pay Rick his salary, but essentially warehouse him as a way of doing damage control with the few good staff he had left.

Over the next few weeks as Frank began the process of picking up the broken pieces of the business, Rick finally sensed how close he was to the line with his father-in-law, who had lost all respect for him. He finally got that Frank was keeping up the pretense for the sake of his daughter and grandchildren, but he felt in his gut that Rick was a loser who he was probably saddled with for life. Rick knew that he must at least give the appearance of seriously trying to get his act together, so he suggested that he attend the dive workshop as a self-improvement and professional development course. He told Frank that he would pay for half the cost out of his own pocket just to show how serious he was about really changing.

Frank looked at the dive workshop Web site and saw that the program was in fact a serious attempt to ignite deep, profound, sustainable change. For the first time he had serious-but-guarded hope that this might actually make a difference in Rick. Rick's main goal for attending was he felt the much-needed break would go a long way toward smoothing things over with his father-in-law. Besides, Rick liked scuba diving, so from his perspective, it was unimportant whether or not he actually got anything tangible out of the workshop and even less important whether he actually changed. Things would work out like they always had if Rick just went with the flow, and at least gave the appearance that he was trying to change.

~~~~~

But Rick can't write *that* on the 3x5 card—what to write? As people begin passing their cards to the head of the teaching table, Thomas silently, and thoughtfully, reads each one. He has cycled through the cards a few times before Rick finally hands in his. Then Thomas begins.

"The main purpose of this setting is to completely remove you from your everyday life. There are no phones, e-mail, TV, laptops or any of the other devices that you use to connect yourself to your everyday world. This setting is like being dropped in the middle of a wilderness, but with all the amenities of home. The location is designed to give you *perspective* on your life. You will view your life back home from a distance. This setting will coerce you to become a spectator of your own life, and becoming a spectator of self is one of the essential elements of deep personal change.

"We will also try to become spectators of self by studying the results of your 360-degree review and Enneagram results on the morning of the second day. The 360-degree review was sent to family, friends, and working associates in order to get a rounded picture of you from the outside in. The goal of the review we do here will be to compare *their* perceptions of you to *your* perception of you and look for significant differences. If your evaluation of yourself is significantly lower than their scores, this may be an area of low self-esteem. If your score is significantly higher, you may have a blind spot in the area probed by that question. We want to identify your strengths and your areas for improvement. The morning of the second day, we will also review your Enneagram results. If you haven't already done so, read the description of your type on the back cover of the RHETI that you were sent, and if you have any questions see me before we do that session."

James raises his hand. Thomas nods and says, "Yes, James?"

"I left my book at home. Do you have another copy I can use?"

"Sure, just see me after the session is over," Thomas says, then addresses the group.

"The boat, while it has all the comforts of home, except for your electronic devices, will create well-defined boundaries. Over the next six days, as we move into the routine of learning, then diving, and spending all of our time within the confines of the boat, the veneer of initial politeness will begin to fray. The boat will become a microcosm, a hothouse that will stimulate insights about you, others on the boat, and people back in your everyday life.

"Every workshop group is different because the people and the life experiences they bring to the table are so varied. The people in this group will bring who they are and where they have been to create the overall mix of the dive workshop experience. Oftentimes, people make deep and lasting friendships here. In a few cases, the dive workshop will become a pressure cooker that makes people feel pretty uncomfortable." Thomas pauses briefly to gauge reactions to this statement. Satisfied, he continues, "The routine of the dive workshop is built around the creative process. Have you ever tried to remember someone's name and you just can't? It's normally when you stop thinking about it, that it just pops into your head. Much of the literature on creativity shows that this is how the creative process works—we apply a sustained effort to learn something or solve a problem, then we stop thinking about it, do something totally unrelated, and that's when the creative insights usually come. This is how I have designed this dive workshop. There will be three fairly intense one-hour workshop sessions each day where we will learn and reflect on deep personal change.

"The sessions will be followed by a dive where you will see some of the most magnificent reefs in the world. As Mike and Kirsten will explain in more detail later, we will limit our bottom-time to sixty minutes because surfacing at about the same time will make it easier to get everyone back on the boat, and limit our nitrogen intake. When we are in Komodo, the nearest decompression chamber is back in Bali, a thirty-four-hour trip by boat.

"My goal is to use the workshop material and the dive experience to purposely *stir up* the unconscious, because the unconscious will process that material and create change, with or without your conscious effort, and sometimes even against your desires. The isolation of the underwater world, where the only thing you will hear is your bubbles, is a great place to have quiet time to reflect. But even if you just put everything out of your mind and enjoy the dive, the unconscious will continue working as part of the creative process.

"As a practical note, some of you may start to have ear problems because you are not used to diving three tanks a day. If this happens, you will have to take your one-hour of reflection time by snorkeling, rather than diving. We will try to arrange the dive sites to where, if people are forced to snorkel, there will be reef structure at about thirty to fifty feet so they can still get a good view of the underwater world here in Indonesia. But I can assure you, snorkeling will not have the same effect as the underwater experience of scuba diving.

"Are there any questions? If not, let's take a fifteen-minute break and then reassemble here so I can review some material that we will need as a foundation for the workshop."

Before Thomas is even done speaking, the steward brings hot cookies and fudge out to the teaching table for a snack. The thing that most people remember about live-aboard dive boats is all you do is eat, dive, sleep, and dive some more. On a regular boat, people can do up to five dives a day. With the dive workshop, there are only three dives during the day, but people can opt to do a night dive after dinner if they want.

Nikki Salem has been sitting in the intense sun getting some color while Thomas was speaking, so she heads down to her cabin to find her suntan lotion. Nikki is tall, slender, with long brown hair and a glimmer of intensity in her flaming, green eyes. Her body is usually restless and in constant motion. She is concerned about the confinement of the boat and how absolutely isolated she is. Occasionally she likes being alone, but most times she wants to be where the action is.

From the time she was a little girl, Nikki was carefree, optimistic and always looked on the positive side of life. She needed constant stimulation, so she would read a book, watch TV, and write a letter to a friend all at the same time. For as long as she could remember, Nikki had the sense that she could not depend on people to give her what she needed, so she had to step up to the plate and meet her insatiable desire for life, experiences, and things by herself. Before she even submitted her completed RHETI booklet, Nikki knew that she was an Enneagram Type Seven, and had been using the Enneagram as a tool for personal growth for some time. Type Sevens are busy, productive people who are playful, high-spirited, and practical. "They can also misapply their many talents, becoming over-extended, scattered, and undisciplined."[8]

Nikki's father was in the military and she had lived more places and had more friends than she could remember. The constant moving bothered her brother Erick, but Nikki loved it. She did her last two years of high school in Sacramento, where her parents finally settled down and where she learned to dive in her first year in college. Nikki had kept in touch with many of the friends she had made, and one of them, Mike, was living on the south side of Manhattan. He invited her to come out and stay with him. With only a few courses to go toward her two-year degree in general studies, Nikki moved to New York in the hopes of finishing school and becoming an actor.

Nikki was always over-committed and trying to do too much, and often let people and tasks alike fall through the cracks of her commitments. Whether it was relationships, school, or a conversation she was having with a colleague, Nikki could not focus on one thing without being distracted by other more interesting things that she feared she would miss out on.

The beat and pace of New York City was a constant stimulation for her. She worked as a waitress in a small French restaurant in Greenwich Village where she learned a lot about wine and food, and three years later she graduated from NYU with a degree in fine arts. Nikki's life was a constant blur of activity as she auditioned for acting parts during the day, waited tables at night, and sandwiched in more social life than most people could handle in a lifetime.

But underneath her smile and happy-go-lucky manner was an inner psychological landscape that was a dry, barren, emotionally parched land. She was a walking oxymoron—she was one of the most accomplished people you would ever meet, but she was also one of the most vacuous people you would ever meet. Nikki could not connect to her experiences in a way that would ground her, so she constantly stayed in motion as a way of distracting herself from experiencing the inner wilderness of her life.

Nikki was never able to make enough money to even marginally support her lifestyle as an actor. She was ready for a change from the humdrum routine of waiting tables and chasing ephemeral parts in second-rate plays, so she took a job in a small publishing company on the Upper East Side where she was able to do everything from editing to marketing and sales. She quickly secured a senior position with the company, and met Todd, who was the lead book editor for fiction offerings. Nikki and Todd moved in together, and at the age of thirty-five, she was the happiest she had ever been in a relationship. Maybe Todd would finally be the one she would settle down with?

Nikki felt that she had to take life into her own hands because life would not naturally unfold for her. She stayed intoxicated with the constant motion of life in the Big Apple and was always planning, looking to the future, mapping out where she was going, who she would be with. Then she would lean on people to try to make reality conform to her plan. Sometimes she pushed ahead so quickly without thinking that she mistook her plan for reality. One of the many guys she dated had once characterized her style as "do-want, push-control." Nikki would say to him, "Let's do this, let's do that, I want this, I want that." When he became overwhelmed by her demands, she would push-control, push-control until he finally gave in and did what she wanted. He always felt like someone with their finger in a human dike that held back an enormous flow of demands. She lost interest in him shortly after she had worn him out both physically and psychologically.

Professionally, Nikki was feeling like she needed a change, so rather than just leave the job as she'd always done before, Nikki applied for an executive MBA program at Yale and just reduced her hours at the publishing company. The train commute to and from New Haven once a week gave her time to read and work on homework, and she was able to use the business aspect of the publishing company as a case study for many of the workshops and seminars she had to write papers on. Nikki had little patience for the realities of what it actually took to get through the MBA program, but it was Todd who had a stabilizing effect on her. When the mundane grind of writing papers or reading books she wasn't interested in, combined with the long commute every week, got her to the point where she was ready to quit, Todd gave Nikki the support she needed to go on and finish. She really loved Todd and wanted the relationship part of her life to settle down, but she knew that once she got her MBA, she would feel the urge to move on to other things.

Nikki was quick on her feet. When one of her professors would ask a question, her hand would first go up, and then she would begin to formulate her answer. Nikki could read the Cliff Notes version of any topic, then instantly pass herself off as an expert in that area. Occasionally, when one of her professors or classmates who really was an expert saw beyond this veneer and pressed her to thoroughly substantiate her opinion or her facts, it became clear that her seemingly endless well-spring of wisdom and knowledge did not go that deep after all. But Nikki would adroitly move on to the next topic or point of discussion. Moving on was her middle name.

Even before she graduated, Nikki was recruited by an international cosmetics company as their field manager for distribution in Europe. In her first year, she was overseas 150 days with no sign that this schedule would let up. While Todd loved Nikki, he didn't want to have to live at this pace for the rest of his life. Todd had heard Nikki discuss the Enneagram and her own compulsion for new experiences often enough that he could see there was no settling down in sight. He discussed this with her over and over again, sometimes on costly long distance calls while she was overseas, and she agreed that she needed to slow down. But Todd knew that she was addicted to staying in motion.

Secretly, she had plans for herself and Todd and she was trying to smooth things over so that she could make these plans happen. Nikki would tell Todd that all she wanted was to be happy with him, but Todd knew that her idea of "happy" was actually a kind of frenetic escapism of which he wanted no part.

Tired of constantly talking with no resolution, Todd began seeing someone else during the time Nikki was away. When he finally told Nikki he was leaving her, she was devastated. It was the first time Nikki had ever been left in a relationship. She had always done the leaving. The break-up with Todd forced Nikki to face herself and what she truly wanted out of life as she had never done before. But even before he left, her discussions with Todd had sparked more pressing inner questions about leaving a legacy with her life. She had been using the Enneagram as a self-help tool, but her biggest challenge was to find a way to stop moving and forever planning out her life, and try to find some inner guidance about how her life should unfold. Nikki came to the dive workshop hoping to find a clear path forward for her life in the wake of Todd's leaving her.

Nikki is no sooner settled in her beach chair on the upper deck when she hears the bell ring for the group to reassemble around the teaching table on the main deck.

As people are getting settled into their places, Thomas speaks, "For the next few minutes, I want to give you a brief overview of the logical geography of the content of the dive workshop.

"The Greek philosopher, Plato, claimed that each of us comes into this world with a destiny—a special calling. We are all meant to do certain things and be someone who is unique unto us. For some people, the calling comes early in life and is like a raging river that they must navigate. We normally associate this type of calling with famous people like Mozart or Einstein.

"But for most of us, the calling is like the quiet flow of a river. During the first half of life it cannot be distinguished from many inner and outer things that clamor for our attention—taking guitar lessons, playing sports, doing photography, and most of all meeting, or rebelling against, the expectations of other people in our lives. Because of the pressure we have early in life to decide, 'What do I want to be when I grow up?' most people automatically equate their *calling* with the question of what they want to do for a living. While it can certainly be about this, the calling I am talking about is 'How do I become the person I am destined to be, but who has never existed?'

"My experience of my own calling has always reminded me of the movie *Forrest Gump* because *destiny* is one of the main themes of the movie. From early on in the film, Gump wonders if he *has* a destiny like his friend Lt. Dan claimed, or whether he had to *create* his own destiny like his Momma said: 'Life is like a box of chocolates, you never know what you are going to get, so you have to make your own destiny, Forrest.'

"As the quiet flow of the river of calling proceeds in the first half of life, the pedestrian realities of our lives convince us that Forrest's Momma was right, we have to create our own destiny. So we occupy ourselves with the tasks of building a life, or more correctly, we spend our time constructing a self." Thomas moves to the flip chart and turns over the blank top sheet to reveal the following chart:

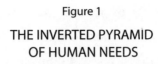

Figure 1

THE INVERTED PYRAMID
OF HUMAN NEEDS

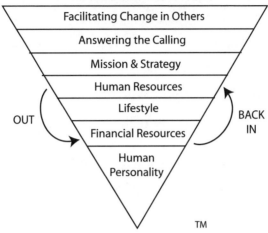

"Figure 1 represents the inverted pyramid of our needs. During the first half of life, if we are lucky enough to have parents who get us through high school and college, we spend our first twelve to sixteen years in school developing ourselves as a human resource that will allow us to assume the responsibilities of adult life. Our overall personality, our gifts and talents, as well as the environment we are raised in, vitally affect how we perform during this time of training. The development of our overall personality is the foundation of all other achievements in life, although most people are not taught to think this way. When we graduate from school, we pop out of the human resource box and are immediately thrown into a world of having to produce money that will determine our lifestyle."

Thomas points to these levels on the diagram, and continues on. "If our desires or lifestyle needs exceed our ability to generate revenue, we can increase the amount of money needed to support the lifestyle we want through installment credit. We can also pursue a long-term solution by getting back into school or learning new skills outside the classroom that will allow us to generate increased revenue over the course of our lifetime. The constant struggle between the demands of lifestyle and our ability to earn revenue dominates most people's lives during the first half of life. This frenetic pace of life drowns out the quiet flow of the higher needs of life's mission, special calling, and facilitating change in the lives of others.

"But for many people who approach the midpoint in life, they have established themselves in the world and have achieved the level of income and assets needed to support the lifestyle they want. As such, their calling becomes louder, stronger, more pressing, more pronounced against the backdrop of their lives. I hear echoes of the calling in some of the 3x5 cards I just read. After the age of thirty-five or forty, half of our time on this one trip through life is gone. We are forced to face the fact that life is a currency that we spend one day at a time, and the question becomes, 'How will I spend what I have left?'

"Your calling is, in part, about living with the consequences of decisions you have made in your lives. But it's much more than this. The calling has a sense of transcendence and destiny about it, and when it begins to press into the fringe of our consciousness, it can create enormous confusion and inner questioning about how we are living our lives.

"Some people come to realize just how tired they are of the daily grind of their professional lives. Others experience an inner restlessness, a hunger for the feeling of meaning and contribution in life, and to leave a legacy. Still others want to begin living a life of authenticity and integrity—the road less traveled. Some people wish they could change, but have no idea where to begin because the calling presents itself like a riddle, or a parable that makes no rational sense. For example, 'I have been working in computing for twenty years, but I don't enjoy it. If I really had a choice, I would quit my job, build a log home in Colorado, get some goats, llamas, and chickens, sew for fun, and stay home and be a full-time mom to my children.' In its most poignant and devastating manifestation, the calling can become a deep and overwhelming sense of desperation where people feel that they have no way out."

To drive home his last point, Thomas reads a story about a woman who lived in the Midwest. "Her idea of a really good time was to board the train to Chicago and wear a big hat, and walk down Michigan Avenue looking in all the shop windows and being an elegant lady. By hook or by crook or by fate, she married a farmer. They moved out into the midst of the wheat lands, and she began to rot away in that elegant little farmhouse that was just the right size, with all the right children, and all the right husband. She had no more time for that 'frivolous' life she'd once led. Too much 'kids.' Too much 'woman's work.' One day, years later, after washing the kitchen and living room floors by hand, she slipped into her very best silk blouse, buttoned her long skirt, and pinned on her big hat. She pressed her husband's shotgun to the roof of her mouth and pulled the trigger. Every woman alive knows why she washed the floors first. A starved soul can become so filled with pain, a woman can no longer bear it."[9]

Bethany Wringer is sitting in the seat that is closest to where Thomas is standing. She is good-looking, with beautiful light black skin and shapely hips and thighs, but wears no make-up and old-style Victorian clothes that give the impression that she is ashamed of her body. Bethany is powerfully moved by the story of the woman who committed suicide because she actually knew someone who had reached this state in her life.

✴✴✴✴✴

Bethany has always been dominated by anxiety, sometimes to the point where people were afraid to tell her things they feared she would worry about. For as long as she could remember, Bethany lived with a nagging sense of inner uncertainty and lack of trust in herself and other people. More than anything, Bethany was ambivalent about life. She had a difficult time deciding how to answer some of the questions on the Enneagram test because she saw some of herself in all the questions, but in the end her score still was clearly an Enneagram Type Six. Type Sixes are committed, security-oriented people who are reliable, hardworking, responsible and trustworthy. They are "excellent 'troubleshooters,' they foresee problems and foster cooperation, but can also become defensive, evasive, and anxious—running on stress while complaining about it."10

Bethany was a caseworker for the Social Services Department of the city and county of Myrtle Beach, South Carolina. She had a passion for helping children who came from dysfunctional families and her job allowed her to do just that. But after a few years, Bethany had become increasingly cynical about the seriousness of the problems she encountered in the families she and her fellow caseworkers confronted every day. What she was unaware of was that her passion and her growing cynicism resulted from her unconscious attempts to use her job as a way to work through her own childhood issues.

Bethany's father, Jerry, was an ultra-fundamentalist preacher who sermonized long and hard about sin and repentance, with a judgmental tone that came through even when he tried to talk about God's love. Her mother, Nadine, was a stay-at-home pastor's wife who had raised Bethany and four other children in a meager country parsonage. They were dedicated to their ministry, and times were often hard. The fundamentalist guidelines and "truth" that Bethany had gotten drummed into her head all her life were what she looked to for guidance in her life, but paradoxically they did nothing to ease her anxiety and worry about this life or the next. If anything, they made things worse. Her parents insisted that she go to a Christian college, and given how well she had done academically in high school, Bethany won a scholarship to attend the Midwest Bible Institute in Chicago, where she studied child psychology.

Bethany found it hard to make decisions, especially ones that had long-term impact. When she finally did make a decision, she would worry herself sick about it and manufacture potential problems that could possibly happen as a result. More than most people, she was dominated by a fear of her ability to survive in life, and she responded to the world reactively and with a sense of urgency and alarm. In the very deepest part of who she was, Bethany lived at the level of her animal instincts, but these could not be trusted because they both detected real danger in life, and also found danger where there was none in a kind of paranoid way. She guarded against this inner and outer uncertainty through a kind of shotgun approach of skepticism toward all of life. Her friends and parents alike knew her to be lovable, friendly and hard-working—the kind of person who would be committed to getting any job done she was given. But beneath this veneer of compliance was a woman who was out of touch with herself in a serious way, and found it difficult or impossible to act independently of the views and opinions of others, because she so thoroughly distrusted her own thoughts and emotions. But at the same time, she would routinely play the devil's advocate with those same people she claimed she trusted.

Her fundamentalist faith became even more calcified at the Midwest Bible Institute, where she was required to sign a doctrinal statement about her faith in God, plus a lengthy laundry list of things she promised not to do while she was at the school. Students were required to attend chapel three times a week, and conservative theology was a significant lens through which all disciplines were interpreted. But compared with the ultra-fundamentalism of her upbringing, Bethany was confronted with defining what she thought about the issues of life and her faith for the first time. The combination of the pressure of schoolwork, her part-time job, and her new freedom stressed Bethany to the point where she began seeing Dr. Paula Jones, a local Christian psychologist. Paula was an open and direct person, and for Bethany, a breath of fresh air. Dr. Jones tried to explain to Bethany that rigid forms of ultra-fundamentalism could be psychologically damaging to people through guilt and manipulation. Many people like Paula still believed in God, but did not have such rigid views. With Paula as her guide, Bethany began to realize that her religious beliefs were creating many of her psychological problems, and to the degree that Paula was able to help her see this, Bethany began the long journey toward freedom from this misplaced religious guilt and bondage.

Bethany met Dave at the Midwest Bible Institute and after graduation they moved back to Myrtle Beach and got married. Dave found a job as the manager of a large hotel and golf course resort. Bethany accepted a position with the Social Services Department. Two years later, they had their first child, whom they named Samuel. After her maternity leave, Bethany returned to work and brought Samuel to the day care run by her father's church where she and Dave attended. One day, she picked Samuel up from day care, drove home, and walked into the hallway of their apartment building where she found Dave and their neighbor Betty talking in the hallway. They weren't doing anything amiss and both Dave and Betty casually greeted her, but Bethany sensed something was going on between them. As they walked to their apartment, Dave explained how he had gotten off of work early that day and just happened to run into Betty in the hallway. Bethany pressed him for answers because her suspicion was running wild. But the more she pressured him, the more he insisted that there was nothing going on between them. It was just a chance meeting and that was all there was to it.

Bethany never took things at face value, and always suspected that there was a contradictory side of the story that was just waiting to reveal itself. In instances when this actually happened, it validated her fears, but ironically it also made those fears deeper and more profound. This inner life of total uncertainty was terrifying to her. But she lacked the courage to begin the journey down what she viewed as the slippery slide that led to facing her *total* uncertainty and inner doubt about all of life, including the fundamentalist faith of her parents. On the rare occasions she had ventured this way, she was horrified about how little she actually knew about herself, her feelings, beliefs, other people and the world. She had almost no confidence in her ability to clearly know and trust her own instincts and even doubted her perceptions about everyday interactions with friends, colleagues, and family. And that's why she soon began to question whether her suspicions about Dave and Betty were fact or fiction. Maybe nothing was happening, and *she* was creating a problem where there really was none.

Bethany had been pleasant, but never friends with Betty previous to the hallway incident. Now there was a wide chasm between them that Bethany could not easily cross. She kept a close eye on Betty constantly, trying to peer below the surface of Betty's life from down the hallway. She found nothing she could put her hands on, but this did not alleviate her suspicion. The lack of hard evidence did nothing to change the way Bethany constantly nagged Dave about this single incident even years later.

Lurking on the fringe of Bethany's consciousness was the hardened belief that people were somehow out to get her, or wanted to undermine her attempts at living her life in peace. Bethany had learned early on that the world was a dog-eat-dog place where people were struggling to survive, most times at the expense of others.

Four years after the hallway incident, Bethany came home from work with Samuel to discover that Dave had moved out. His note said that her non-stop accusations had finally driven him to do what he was being accused of, and that he and Betty had taken an apartment together across town. When she finally called Dave several days later in an attempt to work things out, he again insisted that there had been nothing between him and Betty until very recently, and that it was Bethany's nagging that drove him into Betty's arms.

Dave made it clear that he would have no part of a reconciliation attempt, and Bethany had no choice but to move on with her life. Her parents helped her purchase a small house near the church after the divorce was final, and Bethany set about the task of trying to put this trauma behind her.

That was ten years ago and since that time she'd finished a Masters degree and had turned down a promotion to Department Director because she worried about taking on too much responsibility. At the urging of a close friend, she had taken up scuba diving as both a recreational sport and as a way to meet people, although she was unsure whether she wanted to get into another relationship. She joined a diving club that made frequent trips to the east coast of Florida, which was only a ten-hour drive. Other than Hawaii, Florida was the best diving that the U.S. had to offer.

Because Dave had run off with Betty, her father felt justified in claiming that she had "scriptural" grounds for the divorce and thus could remarry. They were pressuring her to marry another person from their congregation. By this time, Bethany was just about fed up with the ultra-fundamentalist faith and how much her parents had dominated her life. She'd had it with her parents' brand of religion, and had moved on to attend a church that was more open and tolerant. Her parents blamed the liberalism of her psychologist, Paula, and the Midwest Bible Institute for this change in Bethany, but she knew it was a necessary move to maintain her sanity and protect her from a religious framework that would crush her psychologically with mindless, heartless legalism.

On one of the dive trips to Florida, Bethany met a guy named Matt who she really liked. Her parents despised him simply because he went to "that liberal Lutheran Church in the next town over." Matt enjoyed spending time with Samuel, and somehow Bethany felt safe and secure with him, maybe for the first time in her life. They were talking about getting married, but Bethany just wasn't sure. Another couple in the dive club had gone to the dive workshop and just loved it. Given the decisions she was facing with Matt and her crisis of faith, Bethany wanted to go to the dive workshop to try to "clear her head," and get a different perspective on her life. But she did not want to leave Samuel with her parents, and Matt volunteered to watch Samuel so Bethany could go. Matt's generosity further solidified what a caring and supportive man he actually was.

Thomas moves on, "The pressure that the calling puts on us is normally unwelcome because it challenges everything we have come to believe about ourselves and life. What is most disruptive is that these questions come from within us, not from the challenges of people that we defend against in our lives. The net effect is that the calling can, and often does, redirect the flow of our lives like the destructive power of torrents of water that come from snow melting high in the Rocky Mountains. The demanding waves of emotions that come over us and threaten to pull us apart come against our will and despite our best efforts to suppress them.

"Because the first tendency of most people is to associate the calling with outer change, such puzzles either seem unsolvable, or people think they have to dismantle their life in order to answer the calling.

Sometimes dismantling their life works, but most times it doesn't. Some people will do almost anything just to take the pressure off. Typical responses are: 'I need a new job. I need to change professions. I need a new relationship in my life. I need a new house in a new town, in a new part of the country where things are different. I need a new challenge.' Sometimes this *is* what people need, but most times it is not. Most times, outer changes are quick fixes and band-aids. When people make outer changes as a substitute for addressing their inner issues, they almost always take the inner issues with them into the new situation. Not only does the deep inner questioning emerge again, but people often find themselves in situations that are worse than the ones they just left—out of the frying pan and into the fire."

Dan exclaims, "Sounds like a mid-life crisis to me. I would just bear down, keep going, and not let it affect me."

"Yes," Thomas replies. "That's what many people try to do. Unfortunately, the calling has a distinct degree of independence from us. We find ourselves wondering whether it is us or someone else within us that creates the calling. Despite our best efforts to stop it, it comes and goes, but it will not go away permanently. The calling has an autonomy and objectivity within our minds that we cannot control or turn off. Who is it that raises these questions when *we* don't want to hear them anymore? What does it want from us? What are we being called to do? Whatever or whoever it is, the calling comes from a deeper, transcendent place in our psyches. It comes from a mysterious place, not unlike where deeply haunting dreams come from.

"This sense of having *someone else* within us, someone who acts independent of our will, contradicts the common-sense notion most people have that they are a single unified self—the self I call by the name of Thomas. My claim is that this unified self is the person we worked so hard to construct during the first half of our life. For the rest of the sessions, I will call this person we built the *Conscious Self*, the person we labored on for years, the person who agreed to attend this workshop.

"But the independence and objectivity of the calling points to another element in the personality, one that many people only become aware of in the second half of their life. I will call this the *Unconscious Self*. The Unconscious Self is the organizing, harmonizing, unifying force in the personality that stands outside most of our inner conflict like a spectator who looks and watches from a distance. The Unconscious Self has three roles in the human personality. The first role is *to call* us to the life-long journey of discovering a self who was prevented from existing because of inner conflict and duplicity. The second role is *to guide* us along the journey of discovering that unknown self and to allow our true self to emerge in the personality for the very first time. The third role is *to teach* us the wisdom embodied in the Four Competencies needed to answer the calling to discover who we really are." Thomas points to his flip chart and reads the Four Competencies,

1. Know the Depths of Your Personality.
2. Follow the Three Red Flags.
3. Wait for the Synthesis of Opposites.
4. Make Three Commitments.

"The remainder of the sessions are built around these Four Competencies." Thomas pauses as he looks out over faces that are focused on him standing at his flip chart. "So, in the end, Gump's analysis of the paradox of destiny was right when he said that Momma and Lt. Dan were both correct. We *have* a destiny that is defined by the calling of the Unconscious Self and we *create* our own destiny when the Conscious Self works in partnership with the Unconscious Self to walk the path. Are there any questions so far?"

"I just saw that movie again recently," said Nikki. "What Forrest actually says is that the *having* and *creating* of our destiny are both happening at the same time."

"That's right," says Thomas.

Nikki continues, "The whole theme of that movie, as I remember it, is destiny. The opening and closing scenes had a feather floating around in the air, which to me symbolized the question, 'Are we just floating around in life, or do we have ultimate purpose to what we do and experience?'"

"Great insight, Nikki," says Thomas, "That's exactly what I'm talking about. Are there any other questions or comments?"

People who had known Thomas Rose for most of his life characterized him as deep, intense, serious, melancholy, and sometimes depressed—a guy who almost always looked into the dark, uncomfortable dimension of human existence, the parts of life that most people avoided at all costs. Thomas's family was probably more dysfunctional than many of the families his friends grew up in. Somehow these early experiences instilled deep within him a belief that he was not allowed to be too psychologically functional or too happy—life was a serious thing and that should never be forgotten. Partly because of his problematic home life and partly because of how he viewed life, early on, he was often depressed for a year at a time. One day without warning the inner clouds would be lifted, normally because of a new relationship he had started, and then equally without warning the dark, gray, dysfunctional backdrop of his emotional life would snap back into place.

Thomas was raised in upstate New York and earned a degree in philosophy at Columbia by working as a night club entertainer in New York City. Thomas had always been fascinated by scuba diving and to reward himself for making it through college, he went on a trip to the

Big Island of Hawaii to get certified as a scuba diver. This trip and the adventure of diving gave him a new perspective on his life and he became captivated with diving all over the world.

The only thing that Thomas felt he could depend on in life was the understanding he had about life through his own experience. He learned how to trust that experience and learned that he must always be true to himself when that experience showed him something. For as long as he could remember, Thomas was haunted by the question of who he really was. Secretly he was afraid that underneath the surface of life, where it really counted, he had no identity or personal significance, so he was driven to find one inwardly, even if he had to create it and market it to the world.

Thomas was accepted to a graduate program in philosophy at Berkeley, with the hopes of getting a teaching job in a small college or university. To support himself while in graduate school, he got a temporary job at Lawrence Berkeley Laboratory (LBL) as a technician. Given his work at LBL, his interest turned to philosophy of physics and this created a synergy for his graduate studies and his new job. After six months as a temporary worker, he accepted a full-time, entry-level position operating the particle accelerator at the laboratory.

Thomas always had a sense that he was special and had special gifts and a destiny in life, but he really didn't know what that was. What he did best was introspecting, analyzing, reflecting on, and describing his emotions and inner experience. But how does one parlay that talent into a job that someone will pay you to do? He had no idea what the answer was to that question. Thomas was always self-conscious and felt that he was very *different* from other people, *unusual* in some unexplainable way, perhaps weird. As a way of dealing with these feelings, Thomas externalized them in the way he dressed, talked, and the things he did and didn't do. His feelings were so deep and overwhelming that he learned to express himself indirectly, especially through his music and writing. The only way people could actually know him would be to see his image indirectly in a song or a book he had written, a movie in which the characters expressed who he was, or some other indirect self-representation.

Thomas had been in and out of many different relationships, always looking for the ideal partner. When he looked at the relationships that other more "normal" people had he felt a deep sense of envy to the depths of his terminally lonely soul. He escaped the trap of these depressing feelings by reasoning that these were "surface" people who were an inch deep and a mile wide. Of course they would have relationships, but who wanted the prospect of skipping across the surface of life. He was better off being alone, he rationalized, rather than being latched to someone who was only interested in the mundane goings-on of day-to-day life.

One of his many relationships came to an end, and as he was devastated for the nth time, Thomas began to realize how tired he was of this type of personal history repeating itself. He longed to get it right and move on into a deeply satisfying relationship. The break-up with this woman had been more devastating than the others largely because he was so psychologically tired of failure. He began seeing a Jungian analyst named Trina. At the age of twenty-eight, Thomas was sinking down into the black hell of the unconscious, and mapping out what he saw by recording his dreams in a journal. Sometimes he'd paint or draw the confusing or terrifying images that appeared to him nightly. Analysis was a long process of looking under every psychic rock, trekking down every beckoning emotional trail, exploring every archetypal cave that presented itself as an image in some dream regardless how ridiculous or painful it was.

Between the enormous psychological energy that his analytic

process required, the time-consuming projects he was working on at the laboratory, and the two draft dissertations he completed that were rejected, Thomas eventually dropped out of his doctoral program and took a masters degree in philosophy as a consolation prize. Besides his failure at relationships, this was probably the single biggest blow to his fragile self-esteem.

Thomas always had deep intuitions about people, life and things, as if he could see below the surface of the everyday events of life. Thomas could peer into the bizarre, forbidden, unspeakable soft underbelly of human existence, the kinds of things people would hardly acknowledge to themselves even in the quietness of their own soul. He learned the hard way that he should keep these insights, premonitions, and intuitions to himself. On the occasions that he didn't, he was humiliated when people looked at him like he had three heads. He needed time to sort out whether they came from others, or whether they were artifacts of his own complicated experience of himself.

Five years into the analytic process with Trina, Thomas learned the hard lesson that all who travel the road of analysis learn. After you have analyzed every dream symbol, relived the emotions of every traumatic experience in life, turned things over and over in your mind—yes, long after your psychological life has been completely dismantled—the process of analysis leaves you standing there in pieces. After all, analysis is the process of taking apart, and the sad fact is, it comes without a manual on how to put yourself back together again. But by staying with it, Thomas learned that the secret of deep change is that it's something that happens *to* you, not something you do for yourself. In fact, the first and most important step in following the natural process that Jung called Individuation was to stop trying to change yourself and simply wait for the natural process of change to happen within you.

His job at the laboratory and his interest in the social structure of large physics collaborations got him interested in how science was managed. One of his dissertation topics that didn't work out was an analysis of large physics collaborations at Fermilab, another high-energy physics laboratory, about thirty miles outside of downtown Chicago. Thomas began writing and publishing papers on the management of government-funded science and giving invited talks at nationally sponsored conferences, which gave him lots of visibility. With the threat of a 30 percent cut in the U.S. high-energy physics budget, Thomas was laid off. Although this was traumatic, he used the notoriety he had garnered and the connections he had made through his publications and talks to build his own full-time consulting practice.

The consulting world put a different kind of pressure on Thomas than he had previously experienced, but after eighteen years of analysis with Trina, he had learned the final lesson of walking the path toward wholeness. The job of every analyst is to work themselves out of a job, in other words to get you to the psychological place where you can carry on the process of discovering who you really are by yourself.

At forty-seven, when Thomas met and married his wife Grace, the analytic process had taught him that finding his identity lay not in more introspection, but in the simple, mundane realities of life. More than anything, the birth of Thomas's son Mark was the cap-stone on an inner healing process that had taken so many years from the time he started working with Trina. Ironically, Thomas learned that he could only find himself by connecting to and participating in the very things he used to disdain—the realities of life: cooking, changing diapers, chopping wood, and most of all the relaxation that came from scuba diving.

The years of analysis, dream interpretation, and following the deep inner process of the unconscious had transformed Thomas into an intuitive, self-revealing, and authentic person. The resolution of deep inner conflict within the unconscious taught him how to get a handle on his unconscious impulses and to use his insights about himself, life, and other people to help them, especially through his gift of teaching. One of the most valuable lessons he learned through analysis was that the process of discovering who we really are could transform even his darkest experiences into something valuable, that there was meaning and enlightenment in life's suffering.

One of the tools Thomas ran into with his consulting practice was the Enneagram. When Thomas realized that he was an Enneagram Type Four, much of the path that he had walked made sense to him. Type Fours are introspective, romantic people who are self-aware, sensitive, and reserved. "They are emotionally honest, creative, and personal, but can also be moody and self-conscious."[11]

The Enneagram became an enormously powerful empirical tool for describing and predicting people's behavior, including his own. But Thomas didn't understand how to relate the Enneagram to the psychological path he had walked for more than eighteen years as a Jungian. Understanding the power of both systems to raise consciousness and effect personal change, he used them side-by-side and lived in the tension of not knowing how to integrate the two into a single framework.

Over his years as a consultant, Thomas worked with many different organizations, but he became cynical about the probability of real, deep organizational change. The fundamental belief that emerged from this experience was that organizations are composed of individuals, and that they are only changed one person at a time. In frustration, Thomas turned his attention onto the thing that he knew more about than anything else in life, working with individuals who wanted to experience the deep personal change that he had.

The insight of how to integrate the Enneagram and the best of Jung's views came to Thomas after two years of concentrated questioning, study, writing, and teaching on the problem. In effect, Thomas retained the empirical power of the Enneagram in the type descriptions, and replaced the new-age, metaphysical framework espoused by so many Enneagram teachers with his own theoretical framework that had its roots in Jungian psychology. Thomas subsequently developed the material for the dive workshop based on these insights. Thus the dive workshop actually grew out of Thomas's own experience traveling the road of discovering who he really was.

∿∿∿∿

Unlike some teachers, Thomas searches the faces of the people sitting around the teaching table, and waits for people to respond, as if he actually cares if they have questions.

Finally, he begins again. "Okay, I want to ask you a couple of questions. Let's say you head home after this dive workshop and you believe you have really changed, but every person in your world says you haven't and mirrors that back to you, have you really changed?"

Nikki blurts out, "Yes—you have changed."

Thomas turns in her direction and says, "Really. Why do you say that?"

With all eyes focused on her, Nikki thinks about the rationale for her answer. "Well, you can't let other people define who and what you are."

"Okay," Thomas responds, without indicating what he thought of her answer, "What if you believe you have really changed but the inner dissenting voices in your head say you haven't, have you?"

"Yes," Nikki almost shouts, "of course you have."

Like a seamless volley back over the net of discussion, Thomas says, "How do you know that?" This question is more difficult than the first and rather than press Nikki for an answer that she probably doesn't have, Thomas decides to just move on.

"These are tough questions," Thomas smiles, "and I want to present some operational definitions that we will use to navigate these and other questions during the next six days.

"First, everything we know about the world, and I mean absolutely everything, is filtered through the lens of our life and experience, so we never see the world as it actually is. No one here has a 'God's eye view' of truth. Even if there were such a thing as *the truth,* you could not know it without interpreting it through your philosophy of life, beliefs, values, experiences, and all the other things that make up what some have called 'your world view' and what I will call 'your paradigm.' So when we discuss something during the workshop, you will really be comparing your paradigm with others' paradigms.

"Second, since we will not be able to establish the *truth* of situations, we will need criteria for choosing between alternative paradigms, all of which are defendable to one degree or another. For the remainder of the workshop, I want us to use the criterion of *reliability.* Reliability is what scientists look for when they propose theories about how the world works, and then test them over and over again. When a theory passes the test of experiment consistently, the theory is refined to higher and higher levels of accuracy, and becomes increasingly reliable. Eventually scientists come to view the theory's predictive power as law-like, but it never becomes *truth.* So, when I claim that the views presented in the workshop have a high degree of reliability, that means that they can powerfully *describe* and *predict* the behavior and emotional life of people. My views are not *truth,* they are *reliable.*

"Third, we will also need a working definition of what we mean by *reality.* For our purposes, if something is real, it makes a physical difference. If it makes no physical difference, it's not real. In other words, things are *real* if they act on, or interact with, the physical world. Deep personal change must make a physical difference, or else it is not real. This allows us to tease apart the distinction between talk of change, promises to change, intent to change, hoping for change, working toward change, and really obtaining deep personal change. Change must be cashed out, concretized, or otherwise instantiated in the world, or else *it is not real change*.

"Fourth, we need a working definition of what is *objective* and what is *subjective*. When something is objective, it exists independent of the knower. If it does not exist independent of the knower it is subjective. Discussion about the nature of the objective-subjective distinction spans the spectrum of questions from an eight-year-old's fear of thunder and lightning, to the ultimate question about whether God exists. I once explained to a child that while lightning does sometimes hit houses and people, that this is very rare. I then asked her, 'Where is your fear—inside or outside your head?' 'Inside' she said. Her fear is subjective. This distinction is important because things that are *subjective* can be very *real*. The subjective fear of lightning hitting our house can be so real that it causes the child to wake her parents from a sound sleep. So deep personal change can be subjective, but it must be cashed out, concretized, or otherwise instantiated in the world, or else *it is not real change*.

Bethany raises her hand and Thomas turns and faces her. "This happens to some of my clients all the time," says Bethany. "Even when their subjective fears are not based in reality, they become very real and can ruin their lives because the fear makes them act in inappropriate ways."

"That's right," Thomas gestures her way in agreement. "When a subjective fear actually creates problems in a person's life, those problems *become* that person's reality.

"So let's return to my initial question about whether we have really changed if everyone around us says we haven't. In the absence of any objective criteria for choosing between whether we have changed or not, *we must be the final judges* of whether or not we have experienced deep personal change, not the world around us. This statement may raise some eyebrows in the group. I don't know what the basis of your statements were, Nikki, but from my perspective, when we follow this difficult line of questioning all the way to the core, I have found no viable alternative position. If someone in the group can present one, I will abandon this view without a second thought.

"While these assumptions and distinctions help us tease apart the differences between talk of change, promises to change, intent to change, hoping for change, working toward change, and really obtaining deep personal change, we need other *safeguards* to navigate the waters of deep personal change. First, always work on self first and then allow changes in self to influence the aspects of life within which we are embedded. If we go for deep change, these actions will subsequently perturbate outwardly toward the world. Second, we must always be willing to entertain that our view is misguided to the 10 percent level even on the aspects of our reality that we view as unquestionable."

Thomas pauses, looks into the faces of the people around the teaching table and asks, "Now, are there any questions?" There is a silence, even from Dan who always has something to say. "Okay, make sure you use the logbooks that you have in front of you to log your thoughts, insights, and any dreams you might have during the next six days. Keeping a journal is an important aspect of the overall process of discovering who you really are.

"Mike and Kirsten will give the boat debriefing after a short break. I would suggest that you get your dive gear set up if you haven't already done so, so it's ready for our first dive tomorrow morning. Weight belts are over here. If you have any problems with your gear see Mike. For problems with an underwater camera or video unit, see

Kirsten. Kirsten is also in charge of our E-6 film processing lab, which she'll tell you all about during the dive brief. Dinner is at 7:00 P.M. right here around the teaching table on the main deck. The first session tomorrow will begin after breakfast, at 8:00 A.M. sharp, right here."

Lindsey is trying to figure out how many pounds to put on her weight belt. It doesn't seem to make sense that after you've put on an eighty-cubic-foot aluminum tank, your wet suit, and all that other gear, that you would still have to add weight to get you down under the water, but you do. Lindsey debates whether she should use twelve or fourteen pounds. Too little weight, and you will bob around on the surface like a cork and not be able to submerge. Even if you can get down initially, with too little weight you won't be able to stay down at the end of the dive when your air tank is empty and buoyant to the point where it might push you to the surface like a fishing bobber.

Most inexperienced divers over-weight themselves, then compensate by adding air to their buoyancy control device, a BCD, which is the underwater equivalent of the life vests that flight attendants demonstrate how to use on airplanes. The difference is that you inflate your BCD underwater with air from your scuba tank.

People who are inexperienced at inner diving into the depths of the personality often have too much weight—psychological baggage—that they carry through life, threatening to take them below the surface of consciousness. They are forced to compensate for this excess baggage by using psychological energy, which is the most precious resource humans have.

~~~~~

The bell rings at 7:00 P.M. sharp and the group assembes at a table that is covered with a bright blue tablecloth, dinner candles suitably protected from the wind in glass encasings, and a setting of plates and silverware that is as fine as any high-end restaurant in Bali. The steward serves dinner, removes empty plates, and pours whatever kind of wine the guests like.

Most of the discussion focuses on the dives that the group will do tomorrow, how deep they will be, how much current, what the visibility will be like, and what kinds of marine life they are likely to see. Every diver has their own preference for what they like. Some people like seeing "big stuff"—manta rays and the enviable list of hammerhead, gray reef, silver tip, and bull sharks. Other people like the small stuff, paradoxically called macro by underwater photographers. These are the tiny, subtle creatures that only the most observant will ever detect underwater, like pigmy sea horses, cleaner shrimp, sea worms, and nudibranchs that look a lot like sea worms, but aren't. James likes the brightly colored hard and soft coral and the constant activity of reef fish like anthias, butterfly, angel, damsel, and anemone fish.

A few people are discussing with Thomas the material he presented today. For those people who have been on a live-aboard before, this type of serious discussion is not the standard fare. Typically, divers go on these trips to explore the ocean world, and forget about the problems of life for a while. The usual conversations on dive boats focus almost exclusively on diving-related topics. People talk about places they have been diving and how they liked them, what kinds of new equipment they are using and how it performs, what they saw on that last dive, or how that last roll of pictures turned out. It's almost an unspoken rule that other than an occasional side conversation with someone, serious topics are off limits on live-aboard dive boats. But given the purpose of the dive workshop and Thomas' opening remarks, it is clear that serious topics will be the focal point of this trip, and this discussion is designed to enrich the entire dive experience.

It is already 8:00 P.M., and most people have wandered away from dinner to other parts of the boat as it steams its way east toward Sumbawa. Joel, Rick, and Maggie are still sitting at the table even after the steward has removed the tablecloth, revealing the enormous wooden table where the five remaining days of teaching will take place. They can see tiny clusters of lights and some fires on the shore of the island they are sailing across from and they just assume that this must be the island of Lombok. Maggie asks Joel what his favorite dive spot is, and he begins telling her the story of diving the wrecks at Bikini.

Even as a child, Joel Booker's family and friends always viewed him as living in his own little world. He was the "smart kid" in class. As an adult, Joel pretty much knew that when he walked into a room full of people, he would probably be smarter than 95 percent of them, and he took pleasure in this fact. Joel's style was to be an inside-out observer of a world that he never quite felt he belonged in. This was probably why Joel fit in so naturally as a bio-physicist at Los Alamos National Laboratory, the place where Robert Oppenheimer and a secluded and heavily guarded band of physicists invented the atomic bombs that were dropped on Japan. His top-secret clearance meant there were parts of Joel's job that he could not talk about. With a jet-black ponytail, a plaid shirt, and a tweed jacket, in a town that had one of the highest per capita densities of Ph.D.'s in the country, Joel was one of the "coneheads" up on the hill. Like their predecessors during the war years, the Los Alamos scientists were the protected few who kept our nation's defense strong by pouring their creativity and technical prowess into weapons of greater and greater sophistication and destructive power.

Joel didn't put much stock in personality typologies, and ironically when he read the description for his Enneagram Type Five, the intellectual skepticism that is so typical of this type is precisely what made him discard the Enneagram as a waste of his valuable time. Type Fives are perceptive, intellectual, and cerebral people who are alert, insightful, and curious. "They are able to concentrate and focus on developing complex ideas and skills… they can also become preoccupied with their thoughts and imaginary constructs."[12]

His intellectual arrogance and emotional detachment caused serious interpersonal conflicts with his last two secretaries, who filed grievances against him for creating a hostile work environment. His division leader was forced by the laboratory's HR Office to reprimand him and require that he attend a workshop on building his communication and interpersonal skills. Joel viewed this as another kind of "charm school" being taught by a not-so-bright business consultant. When cynically quizzed by one of his colleagues over lunch, "So how was it?" Joel responded, "It was like the revenge of the 'C' students."

It was not that Joel didn't *have* emotions and desires, he hid them from others under a persona of intellectual distance and indifference to the matters of the heart. Joel had become a master at appearing detached and uninvolved when he actually had powerful emotions and desires on issues of life. Rather than take precious time and psychological energy away from his research, if he suspected that his hidden views might cause conflict with someone that he would have to stop and damp down, he didn't give them a straight answer. "Well," he'd say with a long pondering pause, "It's just more complicated than that." That was often the end of the discussion and people never knew where they stood with him.

In the part of his job that Joel could talk about, he had been doing radiation measurement studies in the Marshall Islands for the last twenty-five years. Some of the islands where the U.S. tested nuclear weapons, like Ennewektok, had already been resettled based partly on the scientific rigor of Joel's work. But more than fifty years after the U.S.

removed the natives of Bikini Atoll and detonated thirty-nine thermonuclear devices, Joel and his team of scientists were still studying the radioactive levels of cesium and plutonium on this tiny atoll. In a sense, the goal of the research was to help answer scientific questions about when people could return home. But for Joel, he just loved doing the research and hoped it would go on forever. He had published his results in the top scientific journals, and was viewed as a world-renowned expert in his field. The scientific community had long recognized Joel to be a person with extraordinary technical insight who had charted his own scientific course at Bikini. Joel was able to see the seemingly unrelated connections between the physics problems of residual radiation levels and the biological and environmental problems of vegetation and rainfall levels in this secluded ecosystem.

The isolation of Los Alamos, high on the fingered mesas of northern New Mexico, mirrored Joel's deep need for isolation. Joel always had more research projects than he possibly could handle. He complained about being over-worked and having so little time to relax, but he constantly took on more and more projects as if they were satisfying some insatiable hunger that he had. He worked constantly and was stingy with his time, his emotional life, his psychological energy, and his willingness to meet with and communicate even with his colleagues and associates at the laboratory. His latest secretary, Gena, was under strict orders to protect him from the demands of everyone, even the laboratory director.

The only thing he enjoyed more than his work at the laboratory was his field trips to that isolated speck of sand that rose three feet above the Pacific Ocean, five thousand miles west of California, Bikini Atoll. For over a month at a time, Joel and his team lived in a primitive base-camp that was funded by his research project. Other than a scuba diving concession owned by a businessman in Majuro where Joel had learned to dive years earlier, the base camp was the only thing on the island. The shadowy figures of aircraft carriers, battleships, and destroyers that were brought to Bikini, moored in the lagoon, and sunk as part of the U.S. nuclear testing program, lay on the sandy floor of the lagoon almost two hundred feet below the surface of the crystal clear water. Because of the historical link between Los Alamos and the war in the Pacific, Joel had often done the 185-foot deep decompression dive to see the 780-foot battleship *Nagato*, the boat from which Admiral Yamamoto gave the order to bomb Pearl Harbor. It wasn't that Joel particularly liked wreck diving, it was just that these ships were not "boringly" sunk by airplanes and torpedoes during the war like those at Truk Lagoon. The ships at Bikini are the only ones in the world that were sunk by thermonuclear detonation.

Joel normally felt compelled to debate the merits and shades-of-gray of almost every situation with whoever he was talking to. When he felt pressed for time or psychological energy as he almost always was, he would appear to go along with what his wife or a project leader wanted-ed, but secretly he would just continue to do exactly what he wanted to do and then let them figure it out. Eventually, this type of quiet, iconoclastic, passive-aggressive behavior frustrated and even enraged the most patient of people, which quite frankly was precisely Joel's intent. When people started to understand what Joel was doing, this would only widen the gap between him and other people as they began to question his honesty and integrity.

Joel's house on the hill in Los Alamos was destroyed during the fires of 1999 and this put the final strain on an already problematic marriage to his first wife, Dana, who worked at the laboratory in the HR department, which Joel so thoroughly disdained. After their house was rebuilt in Los Alamos, Dana refused to move back from where they were temporarily living in Santa Fe. Joel's older son was already in college at Berkeley where Joel had gone to graduate school, but rather than endure a long, protracted legal battle over custody of his younger son Robert, Joel reluctantly consented to let him live with Dana in Santa Fe.

For all its intellectual brilliance, Los Alamos had a seedy, almost soap opera side to it where people routinely exchanged significant others and marital partners on an all-too-frequent basis. Within a year of his divorce from Dana, Joel began dating and married Pat, who was the Chief of Staff of X-Division on the weapons side of the laboratory. They immediately had a little girl whom Pat named Sarah. Two years into their marriage, Joel was already having trouble with his wife. Not surprisingly, it was the same kind of interpersonal conflict that he had experienced with Dana.

Joel often substituted thinking about something for actually doing it. In reflective moments when Joel was brutally honest with himself, he knew that this was what he did in his relationship with Pat and Sarah. Intellectualizing his relationship with them was much less threatening than actually having a relationship with them. Joel knew that he should buy his wife flowers once in awhile, take some time off for a family vacation, and spend more time with his daughter who was growing up right before his eyes. But Joel had enormous difficulty initiating action on even the smallest things in life without thinking it to death. At least part of his experience had taught him that if he could just ignore the problems he had in life and stick them into some mental drawer in his mind, six months from now 80 percent of them would no longer be a problem. Unfortunately, Joel would ignore people even when *he knew* they were asking him to do something that was in his best interest. On a practical level, Joel believed that if he could just "stiff-arm" even the legitimate desires of his wife and others for a little longer, most times they would eventually just give up and go away. On the rare occasions that his strategy blew up in his face, he would be forced to stop and do damage control, but this didn't happen too often.

It's not that Joel just "liked" to be alone, his drive for isolation was compulsive. He knew that this caused problems with his first wife and was now causing problems with Pat, but he just couldn't help himself. Joel wasn't a "joiner" or someone who liked to fully enter into things like the dive workshop he was about to attend. His fear of being too involved or sidetracked by anything other than the research projects he chose to work on was precisely why he and Pat were already having serious trouble.

Pat had been pressuring Joel to change, she'd seen the advertisement for the dive workshop in a dive magazine, and thinking that the diving theme was the one way to get him to go, she urged him to attend. Joel initially resisted this intrusion on his research, but when he saw how determined she was for him to start doing things differently, he capitulated and agreed to go. Joel knew that the diving in Indonesia was incredible, but the main reason he agreed to go was in the hope that he might change just enough to prevent this relationship from breaking apart. Another divorce at this time would be a black hole of time, money, and psychological energy that would have to be redirected from his research portfolio.

Nikki is inside the main cabin watching underwater videos from previous trips and looking through the library of books that described the reef life and dive sites they are heading toward. Dan has found a deck chair on the upper deck and is chatting with Lindsey and Bethany about nothing in particular. The moon is about two nights away from being full and the islands they are sailing by have a ghost-like appearance, almost like something out of a dream. They have been in open water for hours and are heading out into a channel between two islands, so the swell of the waves grows larger and pounds on the *Explorer's* bow and occasionally sprays a mist of water that Dan can feel even on the upper deck. The ship dances happily through the water on its way east. It is almost 10:00 P.M. now, and with a big day ahead of them, the divers begin to wander down to their cabins to get some sleep. As Dan lies in his bunk trying to adjust to the motion of the ship, he wonders about Thomas's comment about stirring up the unconscious. What could this mean?

Day 1

DIVING THE REEF OFF SATONDA ISLAND

~~~~~

Competency 1:

Know the Depths of

Your Personality

~~~~~

THE DAY BEGINS

They have sailed all night and in the early morning hours just before dawn, Dan, in a state of
half-consciousness feels the boat stop moving
and the anchor in the forward compartment
begin to drop. They are anchored at Satonda Island, off Sumbawa, east
of Lombok. He can smell the coffee brewing—it is 6:00 A.M. and James
is still sleeping, so Dan quietly gets dressed and heads up to the main
cabin for breakfast.

Most people don't sleep well the first night on a live-aboard
because of the constant motion of the boat moving through the water
and the sound of the waves slapping against the hull two feet from
their heads. As Mozart plays softly in the background, people keep
straggling in for breakfast, comparing notes on how bad their first
night of sleep was. But after the rigors of diving three or four tanks
the first day, the motion and sound of the boat at night becomes a
non-problem as people fall asleep from a deeply satisfying experience
of physical exhaustion.

They are anchored in a small bay, and the magnificent colors of the
water over the reef are visible from the upper deck where Dan is stand-

ing. On the beach there is a white man-made arch of some sort, which is interesting because the island looks deserted. Dan looks east at the shadowy figure of a twin-peaked mountain that Mike said over breakfast was the volcano they would dive near on the last day of the trip.

Thomas is out on the deck furiously writing notes on his flip chart, trying to ready himself for the opening session. He has turned the main deck of the dive boat into a classroom, all centered around the teaching table. Thomas wanders over to the main cabin and sticks his head inside. "We're going to get started." Then he rings the bell that signals the beginning of the first session.

SESSION 1: AM I JUST ONE PERSON?

"We live in the three-pound universe between our ears, but it is amazing how little we know about ourselves," Thomas begins. "Today's sessions will cover the first of the Four Competencies I mentioned yesterday, which is to enable us to gain a deeper understanding into the totality of our personality.

"I want to return to one of the issues we discussed yesterday, which is our natural tendency to experience ourselves as a single unified whole. Most of us have simply adopted the unquestioned intuition, 'I'm in here and the world is out there.' The *I* is the person who has opinions, beliefs, favorite foods, and the strategies and knowledge for getting through life. It is this *I* who has had all our experiences in life, the one self, the *me* who has become what I call the *Conscious Self*.

"But if we hold to a single, unified sense of our personality, how can we explain the experience of saying we are going to do one thing, but end up doing the exact opposite, even though *we* didn't want to? How can we explain the fact that we can't change our emotions because so often they have us, rather than us having them? How can we explain making a commitment to a person, project, or activity, and then our psychological energy goes south and something inside us refuses to keep the commitment? How do we explain the experience of *fringe consciousness* and creativity where ideas, insights, and creative solutions just come out of nowhere? How do we explain the objective independence of *the calling* if we insist on holding on to a unified sense of personality?

"The *central claim* of this session is that the human personality is not a single unified entity. Rather, it is an interrelated system of competing and conflicting elements that must be organized, harmonized and unified into one integrated whole. In order to illustrate this, I want to use a two-part thought experiment to describe the nature of our personality.

"In the first part of the thought experiment, let's imagine that you are the president of a small company. As president, you have bottom-line responsibility for the company and can issue policies and procedures for how you want the company run, but you don't have direct control over the emotions, desires, and wills of the people in your company. These people are *objective* and independent of you, the president, in the sense we defined objective yesterday. In other words, your employees exist, independent of you as president. In addition, your employees are *real* in the sense that they make a physical difference to the company, and what they do determines whether you fail or succeed as a business.

"In the second part of the thought experiment, I'd like you to turn your introspective eye within. Imagine that I am the president of the Thomas company, and you are the president of the Lindsey or Joel company, but that the corporate facility is your body and what is done with that facility is what you do with your life—how you spend your one trip through it.

"Now imagine that you have people in an inner company who occupy that facility, and although you want to run your life a certain way, you do not have direct control over the emotions, desires, and wills of these Inner People. They have their own little personalities, values, goals, and philosophies of life and some of them are diametrically opposed to yours as president. You want to slow down and work less hours, they want to drive on. You say you love your wife and family, they want to leave. You say you need to stay on a budget, they go out and buy a new car. But what is most problematic is that these Inner People are every bit as objective and independent of you as the people in an actual company. The Inner People are objective in the sense we defined above, they exist independent of you the president."

Lindsey sits forward in her seat and says, "Thomas, is this like having different *sides* to your personality?"

"Yes, it's something like that, but the Inner People I'm talking about are more than *sides* to a single, unified personality. The Inner People are like many different personalities all within the multiplicity of your personality."

"So are you suggesting that we all have multiple personalities?" Lindsey asks in disbelief.

"Yes, in a sense," Thomas replies. "I am suggesting that having a multiplicity of different personalities in each of us is a normal, psychologically healthy phenomenon that we all experience to one degree or another." Thomas walks closer to Lindsey's side of the table and faces her directly. "If we were *abnormal* psychologically, we would have these different personalities within us, and would move from one to the other and not be aware of it. Such people are normally diagnosed as having a Multiple Personality Disorder. *Consciousness* about the presence and activities of the Inner People is the difference between being categorized as *normal* or *abnormal* psychologically."

Lindsey's eyes are wide as she and some of the others nod, showing eagerness to know more.

Thomas continues, "To put it another way, your Inner People exist in a virtual state and they only become real when they take over your facility, because only then can they make a physical difference. You say you're going to be nice to your employees, and one of the Inner People grabs hold of the *microphone*—your vocal chords—and hammers them verbally, and you don't even realize it till after the fact. Or one of the Inner People takes over your facility and grabs your credit cards and goes shopping when you just swore that you would stop spending. When the Inner People have charge of your facility, they can control the way you talk, what you do, how you feel, where you go, and how long you stay. What they do when they have control of the facility can vitally affect the course of your life. The Inner People can make or break you, just like employees can make or break the president of a real company.

"Most of the Inner People are psychologically and socially under-developed because they have been locked away in the unconscious and have not been given much facility time. The Inner People are like a child who has been locked in a closet for the first part of his or her life and when they get control of your facility, it's like finally breaking out of this inner prison. No wonder they are so problematic!

"Imagine that some of the Inner People routinely confront you as president and force you to give up control of the facility, which is essentially to force you to give up control of your life. You are aware of these challenges to your authority and you have to deal with them all the time. Some of the Inner People are overt about their activities, others exist only on the fringe of your consciousness. Sometimes, you as president have tried to be open to the desires of the Inner People, especially when you are at introspective workshops like this one. But then the Inner People demand things that change or disrupt your life, so you shut them down with a brutal, survival-type response. They simply retaliate and try more covert tactics to take charge of the facility—and the battle rages on for a lifetime.

"All of your life you have had to manage and control the duplicities and opposing forces of this group of inner insurgents, and prevent them from ruining your life. You probably have succeeded at this fairly well, but it has cost you an enormous amount of psychological energy, energy you've squandered on damping down the inter-office politics of this rag-tag group of people who live within you."

Thomas walks back toward the flip chart, turns to face the group, stands there for a few moments of silence, then says, "Here is the most radical implication of the model of the Inner People. The turbulent emotions associated with this inner conflict belong to the Inner People, but we experience them as *our* emotions, not theirs. We experience their emotions as ours because we all live in the same body and because most of us have a unified view of the personality, so who else's emotions could they be? Maintaining a unified view of our personality requires us to *fabricate* reasons why we have so much inner conflict. For example, if you are an easygoing person and one of the Inner People grabs the microphone and gets up in someone's face, maintaining a unified view of personality forces you to fabricate explanations for our behavior. 'I must be under stress. Maybe I'm depressed. I must be having a mid-life crisis. I must not have gotten a good night's sleep. You must have set me off. I must be grumpy because I'm hungry. I must be feeling insecure.' We fabricate the most fantastic stories—anything to preserve the myth that we are a single, unified self.

"As we approach the second half of life and we begin to experience the calling of the Unconscious Self, this only adds to our inner confusion because it becomes one more set of inner forces that pull us in still different directions. We have to fabricate even more stories to explain why we don't really know what we want to do with our lives.

People have a difficult time answering questions like, 'What do I want out of life?' because they try to act *alone* in the psychological universe of personality that has many powerful players. These people should be asking, 'What do *we* want out of life?' It is the emotions of the Inner People and the calling of the Unconscious Self that we experience as our own and that leads us to feel like spectators in our own minds.

"I'd like you to reflect on two questions between now and the next session. First, 'How well does the model of the Conscious Self, the Unconscious Self and the Inner People explain my inner experience?' Second, 'How can I give the Inner People more facility time so they can become a *real* factor in my life in the sense of making a physical difference?' Make sure you log any insights about the material or your dive in the logbook we handed out yesterday.

"Are there any questions or comments?"

Most people will need time to formulate their questions and they are eager to get into the water where they will have time to think and reflect on what Thomas has said. Other people do not want to discuss their questions in front of the whole group so they wait to chat privately with Thomas after the session is over. Nevertheless, after each session Thomas likes to set aside a time for those who want to discuss the material with the entire class present.

"Okay, this first dive will be a check-out dive so we can make sure of your buoyancy control and adjust the amount of weight you're wearing. It will also give Mike and Kirsten a chance to get some sense of the level of your dive skills. Let's gear up while Mike gives us the dive brief on this site, which is called the Bay Entrance of Satonda Island."

The crew loaded the divers' gear onto two twenty-foot tenders that had been hoisted onto the top of the main boat for the trip over.

The first boat was for people who had underwater cameras and video equipment, and Kirsten was the dive instructor for this group. The second boat was for everyone else, including Thomas and Mike. One by one they stepped into the tenders from the stairs leading down from *Explorer's* port side, then the boats headed for the dive site, which was directly off the arch on the beach.

The procedure was to get your gear on, then your fins and mask, and sit up on the edge of the boat. When Mike and Kirsten gave the signal, they would all roll back off the boat into the water. It takes a few seconds to get your bearings when you first hit the water and begin falling below the surface. Joel always checked his gear: were his two dive computers activated? Was all the air out of his Buoyancy Control Device (BCD)? Was his mask on properly? Was everything else working? Although Mike and Kirsten had told everyone that they needed to pick a buddy to dive with, Joel never dove with a buddy. He preferred diving alone. Besides, he didn't want to have to risk his own life to help save someone from a diving problem just because their competency level was inadequate. He told Mike and Kirsten that he would just buddy up with the group rather than one particular diver, and they said they would only agree to this after the checkout dive. The other divers were waiting on the surface with the group. Lindsey had decided to go with twelve pounds and couldn't get down, so she had to go back to the tender and clip another two pounds on her BCD.

As Joel, Thomas, James, and Dan hung about twenty-five feet below the surface of the water waiting for the rest of the group, the underwater world exploded in an overwhelming visual buffet of color and life. The visibility was easily one hundred feet horizontal underwater. One by one as the group dropped below the surface of the water, Mike and Kirsten gave each diver the hand signal that asked them, "Are you okay?" and each diver signaled back. Within the first fifteen minutes of the dive, they already had a sense for each diver's ability. Buoyancy was the dead give-away. Did they just float effortlessly in the water as buoyantly as the fish and use their fins only to propel themselves forward, or were their hands waving and their fins bicycling to try to maintain their position in the water? Buoyancy is one of the key dive skills to master because the laws of physics are quite different underwater. Water is eight hundred times more dense than air. Objects look 25 percent closer underwater, and sound travels four times faster underwater than in air. Good buoyancy skills get you, "out of your head and present to your body," because buoyancy is something that you sense by the movement of your body in the water. About twenty minutes into the dive, Mike and Kirsten looked at each other with relief, because, while there was a variety of dive skill levels in the group, they all appeared like they'd be able to handle the diving they'd be doing over the next five days.

Thomas was always overwhelmed by the beauty under the water's surface. He hovered motionless over an enormous red carpet of anemones watching a family of clown fish dart in and out of the protection of poisonous tentacles that would harm other fish. As he watched the drama of the clown fish family unfold, the notion of the objective nature of the unconscious intermittently pressed its way into Thomas's consciousness. This insight had always been the most fundamental insight for Thomas, without which the other parts of building the theory and practice of the dive workshop would not have been possible, or made sense. During the years when he lived under the tyranny of being just one person, no wonder Thomas was dominated by the emotional roller coaster, melancholy, and depression he experienced. Until he realized that these powerful inner forces belonged to the Inner People, *not him*, and until Thomas could stand back from his years of identifying with these emotions as his own, he could never be free of the prison that had held him since childhood.

SESSION 2: WHO IS IN CHARGE OF OUR PERSONALITY?

It's 11:00 A.M. and Thomas rings the bell to start the next session. By the time he reaches his flip chart, the last few people are taking their seats. "I want to give you a heads up. This will probably be the most *theoretical* session of the entire dive workshop and the one that is most likely the hardest for you to connect to experientially, at least initially, so ask questions, and try and stay with me, Okay?" A chorus of "okay" and "yeah" issues from the divers.

"If the human personality is really an interrelated system of competing and conflicting elements, who's in charge of the personality? In answer to this question, the *central claim* of this session is that *no one* is in charge of the personality. Our experience tells us that the human personality is more like an inner civil war where the Inner People battle to gain total control of the personality at the expense of other psychic elements."

Thomas gives Bethany two drawings to pass around the table. "I want to talk about a three-level model of the personality that describes: a) the origin and development of personality, and b) structure and workings of the human personality. I believe this three-level model describes and predicts our behavior and inner experiences better than the unified view does, and even goes beyond to describe the deepest things we know about ourselves and the world around us. The three-level model echoes many of the views of Carl Jung, but would probably not be considered classical Jungian thought." Thomas flips a page and gestures at the following chart:

Figure 2

THE HUMAN PERSONALITY

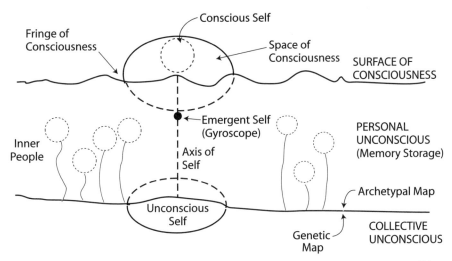

TM

"Let's begin by discussing the origin and development of the personality as shown in Figure 2. Discussions about the origins of the personality are essentially about the nature-nurture question. In other words, to what degree am I who I am because I have genetically inherited tendencies (nature), and to what extent have I been socialized to be the way I am (nurture)? If you side too closely with the nature side of the equation, you risk losing a sense of people having the free will to choose in life. If you side too heavily with the nurture side of the equation, you have a difficult time explaining the growing evidence that many aspects of our personality are passed on genetically from our parents. The view that I find most persuasive includes a major contribution from both sides of the nature-nurture equation. In other words, much of the fundamental pattern of our personality is defined along the biological-psychological interface, and the exact form that this pattern takes depends on the environment we are raised in.

"Figure 2 shows the three levels of the human personality. The first level is consciousness, which I define as a psychological space in the human brain within which we are inwardly aware of, and present to, whatever resides there. Like the RAM memory of a computer into which we load programs, consciousness has no mental contents of its own. Whatever appears in that space, we are aware of *right now*.

"The second level is the personal unconscious that is the enormous memory storage locations in the human brain. When you are able to recall your mother's name, the title of your favorite song, or the name of your second grade teacher, this information is retrieved from memory locations in the personal unconscious. Until these bits of knowledge are summoned into the space of consciousness, they exist, but we are not aware of them.

"The third level is the biological-psychological interface of the Collective Unconscious that is like two sides of a coin. The biological-psychological interface is the place where the hamburger you ate for lunch, becomes the inspiration to develop a new marketing plan, redesign your living room, or any other of life's tasks. On the biological side of the coin, the interface contains the *genetic map* that helps determine who we will become *physiologically*. The psychological side of the coin, called the collective unconscious, contains the *archetypal map* that helps determine who we will become *psychologically*. In the same way hunger, thirst, the herd instinct, and the desire to procreate are different manifestations of biological reality, the archetypes are different manifestations of psychological reality. At birth, the archetypal map already defines the overall psychological structure of our personality. The specific concrete nature of that structure is defined by our experiences in the environments we grow up in."

James says, "My son Jon is only seven months old and he already has a recognizable personality. In your view, his archetypal map is already defining the overall structure of his personality, is that correct?"

"Yes," Thomas says, "the combination of his archetypal map and the environment you are raising him in, are both happening together just like Forrest's view that having and creating a destiny are both happening together at the same time."

Most of the people in the group have their heads down, writing furiously in their logbooks.

Thomas continues, "Prior to birth, children are merged with the mother into one unified whole. Birth is an enormous shock because consciousness is flooded with sense data, and newborn babies do not know what these mean. They hear a sound and are unsure if they should be scared, or happy. The child still has no sense that he or she is a distinct being and has an objective, independent existence apart from the mother.

"As the organizing, harmonizing and unifying element in the personality, the Unconscious Self begins the life-long process of the growth of the personality by allowing part of itself to rise into consciousness, with the goal that the child will come to understand that it is objective and independent from the mother."

Thomas points to the diagram, "As Figure 2 shows, the Unconscious Self extends an Axis of Self up into the space of consciousness. Like the flower of a rosebush that is distinct from, but ultimately connected to the roots of the plant deep underground, the development of multiple psychic entities is part of the natural process of the growth of the human personality.

"But this begins the battle for consciousness because the archetypes that make up the archetypal map also want to occupy the space of consciousness. Like puppies who compete for their mother's milk, the archetypes are hungry and thirsty for access to the world of consciousness, which is the only way they can become real, the only way they can make a physical difference in life. This not only requires that the archetypes occupy the space of consciousness, but that they have control of the facility.

"As the archetypal map of the personality unfolds, the portion of the Axis of Self that occupies consciousness begins to accumulate experiences, associations, and emotions that possess psychological energy. These energetic experiences begin to cluster around the central archetypal core like the individual strands of a ball of yarn and this grouping of experiences becomes what Jung called a complex. The combined psychological energy of the experiences that make up the complex acts like a magnetic field that draws even more energetically charged experiences to itself. Eventually the complex develops preferences for attracting only certain kinds of experiences. Experiences that are interpreted as creating fear, anxiety, or confusion are not allowed entrance into conscious awareness. Some of the rejected experiences register in the unconscious, others don't register at all. This complex of feelings, experiences, associations, and emotions that results from the Axis of Self occupying consciousness becomes what I have called the Conscious Self."

"So the Conscious Self is just one of many complexes that eventually form in the personality, is that correct?" asks Nikki.

"Exactly." Thomas begins to pace back and forth in front of the flip chart and the group resonates to the intensity of his body language and his words. "The other archetypes also struggle to occupy consciousness so they can become real, and likewise become complexes. These other complexes become what I call the Inner People. By design, the Conscious Self begins to dominate the space of consciousness and becomes more and more powerful at the expense of the Inner People, who are forced to develop psychologically in three ways:

"First, the Inner People can still succeed in occupying the space of consciousness during the first few years of the child's life, as they become complexes. They too develop preferences that filter out experiences, associations, and emotions that create fear, anxiety, and confusion for them. Eventually, these Inner People take on lives of their own as semi-autonomous, objective little personalities within our overall personality.

"Second, because the Conscious Self has increasing control over access to consciousness, it is able to filter out experiences that create fear, anxiety, and confusion for itself and becomes the gatekeeper of conscious awareness. But the magnetic attraction of the Inner People in the unconscious draws some of the experiences rejected by the Conscious Self to themselves. For example, if you have lunch with your mother, this experience might result in a total of one hundred different experiential elements. The Conscious Self might select only ten of these elements based on its preferences. Some portion of the other ninety experiential elements is attracted by, and becomes part of, one of the Inner People that we'll call the Mother Complex. Those aspects of the experience of 'having lunch with Mom' that are drawn to the Mother Complex become the *other side of the story* about Mom, and may reveal a contradictory or fundamentally different view of Mom than the one held by the Conscious Self. For example, something in her body language, what she says, or how she said it may come from one of Mom's Inner People who hates and resents you for having been such a burden on her life—feelings she may be largely unaware of, or never admit to you.

"Whether it is a business associate who is intimidated by you, a friend who wishes she had married your husband, or a neighbor you talk to periodically who is jealous about how nice your house is, the other side of these stories register in your personal unconscious as valuable information. This view of the person is often contradictory to the image that your Conscious Self has about them, and the other person may only be marginally aware of these feelings because they exist only on the fringe of their consciousness. Have you ever sensed that people are not what they seem, they are not to be trusted, they really don't mean what they say, they really don't care about you as much as they say they do? Often this is how we experience the activity of *their* Inner People—parts of their personality that they may be totally unaware of. This is why we should believe what people *do*, not what they *say*—often the other side of the story in relationships only comes to light by watching what people do.

"The third way the Inner People are forced to develop is by pressing their way into the fringe of consciousness and gaining some access to experiences that give them increased levels of psychological energy."

James raises his hand and Thomas acknowledges him with a nod. "I have always learned to trust my gut level intuition and response to people and situations, even when they are so radically different from what my other experiences of that person have been. I've always regretted the times I went against my gut because those intuitions have always turned out to be right. What I've been calling *gut intuition* all these years, isn't that what you're calling 'the other side of the story' that comes from the contradictory actions of the Inner People in others?"

"Exactly," Thomas responds. "There's nothing mysterious about this kind of gut level instinct and intuition. The Inner People are a real part of you and are constantly gathering information about life and experiences that never register in consciousness. The repository of knowledge of the Inner People is an enormous asset that we have in life, but most people ignore or silence the signals that the Inner People send when they press into the fringe of our consciousness. People often have much more knowledge than they are willing to act on, because they have never learned to listen to and trust their gut level instincts and intuitions. Regardless of what you call it, sounds like James has learned to tap into and trust the inner knowledge I'm talking about. Any other questions?"

James is busily marking some notes in his logbook as Thomas moves on. "By the second or third year of the development of the child's personality the Conscious Self has displaced the majority of the space of consciousness and, in addition, it is storing more and more of its experiences below the level of consciousness. As the battle for consciousness rages, the Conscious Self gathers a high enough level of psychological energy to give it an almost exclusive hold on consciousness and an enormous amount of memory storage in the personal unconscious. At this point in personality development, three things happen:

"First, the complex of feelings, experiences, associations, emotions, and preferences of the Conscious Self dominate consciousness so powerfully and so consistently, the child experiences them as his or her own, rather than as belonging to only one of many complexes in the human personality. For all intents and purposes, from this time on the Conscious Self becomes the *center of consciousness* in that there is no experiential difference between the Conscious Self and the child. They become identified in the sense that the Conscious Self becomes the only self we know well into the first part of life.

"Second, the Inner People are increasingly prevented from entering consciousness so they try to undermine the Conscious Self's control of consciousness by either taking over the facility, or pressing their way into the fringe of consciousness in the hopes of dominating the space of consciousness.

"Third, the Conscious Self becomes inflated and intoxicated with its own power and increasingly loses touch with its origins in the Unconscious Self. This is experienced as an *alienation from self* and the feeling that something very fundamental has *been lost*, or *gone wrong* in life.

"Now with almost unlimited access to consciousness, the Conscious Self spends the first half of life learning problem-solving skills and strategies from parents, friends, TV, books, movies, and personal experiences. When the Conscious Self goes to school, college, grad school, these skills are exponentially increased and honed to a fine edge. The success of the Conscious Self in manipulating life and achieving its own goals provides powerful empirical evidence that the Conscious Self *is* the only psychic element in the human personality.

"As I just mentioned, the Inner People have very different sets of data and problem-solving skills from the Conscious Self. The Unconscious Self has a still different, archetypal perspective that is anchored in the ancient human experience and knowledge of the Collective Unconscious. Consequently when we ask a question such as, 'What is my destiny in life?' the Conscious Self, Inner People, and the Unconscious Self all give fundamentally different answers to the same question. We experience these different, and sometimes contradictory, responses as psychological confusion about what we want and where we're going in life."

"So if we adopt your view," Dan comments, "most of who we are is below the surface of consciousness."

"That's right," says Thomas, again pointing to the chart. "The totality of the human personality is shown here in Figure 2. The warring interaction of all these parts of the personality are precisely why it is not possible to have a single *someone* in charge of the personality. The ongoing battle for consciousness, combined with a tendency to hold onto a unified sense of personality, has two major consequences.

"First, the battle prevents the organizing, harmonizing, and unifying function of the Unconscious Self from operating within the personality. With a unified view of the personality, most people mistakenly attribute their inner conflict as resulting from other people, the world around us, or the biological dimension of the body (which is partly true, but not the whole truth). Consequently, the personality remains fragmented by inner civil war.

"Second, the natural product of the integration and wholeness of the personality should be what I will describe later as the Emergent Self. The Emergent Self rises out of the wholeness and integration of the personality where the whole of the personality is greater than the sum of the warring parts. But the inner civil war and the belief in a unified personality prevents the Emergent Self from coming into existence. The end result of the process of self-discovery is to become the self we were destined to be, but never were, the Emergent Self.

James raises his hand, "Thomas, can you back up and help me understand the difference between the memories and strategies that the Conscious Self stores in the personal unconscious, and the memories and strategies of the Inner People?"

"Of course, James," Thomas grins. "The Conscious Self uses the personal unconscious as a database to store memories and experiences that cannot all be kept in consciousness. Memories get recharged with psychic energy whenever they are brought into consciousness. Frequently used information is stored in memory locations that are easily accessible. Information that is not used as frequently and that begins to lose psychological energy sinks to memory locations that are further and further from the reach of the Conscious Self's retrieval mechanisms. Once these memories fall to a low-enough level of psychological energy where they are no longer accessible to the Conscious Self, they continue to exist, but we experience this as *forgetting* something. Memories that have been forgotten can be re-energized and raised to more accessible memory locations if they are brought to consciousness once again. Experientially, we call this *remembering* something.

"Let me give you an example. I received a notice that my high school in upstate New York would be holding our twenty-year high school reunion. Since I had moved far away from my hometown and had almost no contact with anyone from high school, nor had I attended previous reunions, I decided to go. After twenty years, I had little or no memory of most of my schoolmates, even though I had spent significant amounts of time with them twenty years earlier. I flew back to my hometown a few days prior to the reunion and stopped by my old high school to pick up a high school yearbook from 1970 in the hopes that it might 'jog my memory' about my schoolmates. As I sat in the high school parking lot near where I used to board the school bus, I began to leaf through page after page of pictures of faces that I had once known. By the time I had reached the end of the book, I recognized a number of the faces, and began to leaf through it another time. This time additional faces became familiar once again, so I did it a third time which revived still more memories and faces. I began to question whether some of these people were only known to me by sight, or whether I actually had relationships with them. At the reunion dinner party that occurred a few nights later, I realized how many of these people I had actually known and 'hung out' with. They told me stories about myself that I had forgotten, and memories about them emerged in my mind that they had forgotten. Some of us that had been schoolmates since grade school went out after the dinner party and shared old and new memories until 5:00 A.M. It was like we just did not want to leave.

"This entire reunion experience gave me new insights into the nature and workings of the personal unconscious. The process of looking through the high school yearbook, the dinner party, and the late night discussions gave me a deep and enormously profound sense of having *reclaimed a lost part of myself* that had been long gone. It gave me a sense of rootedness, an understanding of my personal history, and helped me make sense of various aspects of my life. I will never forget it. But it has been twelve years since I have been to the reunion and I have spent almost all of that time living on the Big Island of Hawaii, sixty-five hundred miles away from my hometown. Most of the names, places, and memories of my schoolmates have once again fallen back into the unconscious. Even the experiences that I had with them only twelve years ago at the reunion have faded from memory and cannot be easily retrieved."

Thomas walks to the other end of the teaching table where James is sitting. "But I want to directly address James's question about what the distinction is between the memory storage of the Conscious Self and the Inner People. The fact that I was able to reclaim the high school memories shows that they were not aspects of my life experience that the Conscious Self sought to censor. If they had been, they would have existed as the memories of the Inner People and might only have been able to press into the fringe of consciousness. If they had been the memories of the Inner People, the Conscious Self would not have allowed them to become conscious so easily, or at all. The Conscious Self's strategy for censoring the memories of the Inner People from consciousness is simply to deny them the recharge of psychological energy that they get from being in consciousness. By denying them psychic energy, the Conscious Self tries to exterminate, starve, and ultimately kill the mental contents of the Inner People. But these lost parts of our experience (pleasurable and painful) are part of the totality of who we are, and are never totally lost to us. They may sink to a low energetic level in the unconscious like the ship Titanic, and exist in the silence and unknown darkness of the ocean floor of the unconscious. But the Unconscious Self can, and does, cause these images, memories, and the Inner People to appear on the fringe of consciousness, or as symbols in our dreams that penetrate consciousness. When we consciously take note of these psychic elements for the first time by writing these insights and dreams down and letting them integrate into consciousness, they are raised to new levels of psychic energy *despite* the best efforts of the Conscious Self to the contrary. Having been infused with psychic energy, the memories and activities of the Inner People, which we have never been conscious of before, become accessible because they are moved to levels of the unconscious that are easier to access from consciousness. Does that get at your question, James?"

"Yeah," James says.

"Are there any other questions?"

James looks like he is going to ask another question but changes his mind. James is bothered by Thomas's claim that the Inner People are objective and independent of him, and the fact that his control of the personality is an illusion. The independence of the Inner People does explain his intensified experience of being taunted by his past, by a vengeful, abusive self, who is intolerant to the feelings of others. He just can't stop those inner voices, so he knows he can't have total control over the personality. It is James's deep sense of spirituality that allows him to peer into the place where some of his deepest conflicts and weaknesses are. Behind his seemingly impenetrable walls of strength and power is one of the Inner People—a needy, clingy child who wants more than anything to he held, nurtured, and cared for. James has a vested interest in not letting this Inner Person take over his facility and fights it back at every turn. As Thomas talks on, James feels this Inner Person press into the fringe of his consciousness. Like his seven-month-old son, Jon, this Inner Person is a weak, insecure, helpless, dependent little child who is demanding that James get close to people, love them, be emotionally intimate with them and trust them. James has experienced this intrusion into consciousness before but has always brutally forced it out of conscious awareness. This time James allows this Inner Person to stay and endures the psychological threat and enormous inner pain that acknowledging this long-repressed part of his personality brings with it. How can he ever acknowledge this experience of himself to another living soul without risking more than he is willing to give to any other human being?

Thomas continues, "The Conscious Self does not acknowledge the other psychic elements because it views them as a threat to its totalitarian control over consciousness. Insisting that the Conscious Self is all there is to the human personality is like insisting that the tip of the iceberg is all that there is to the overall iceberg. Each of you has the three psychological levels shown in Figure 2, but most people are only aware of the center of consciousness—the Conscious Self. There is a lot to the saying that even the brightest of us, like Einstein, only have access to, and use of, 10 percent of our brain.

"To use another analogy, the totality of the present scene should include the ship we are on, the reef structure, and the deep blue ocean, but all we are aware of sitting here on deck is the perspective of the part of the ship that is above the water. We know that these other elements of the scene are here, but we are not conscious of them at this time." Thomas walks back to the flip chart, pauses, flips the page, then points to Figure 3:

Figure 3

THE PRESENT SCENE

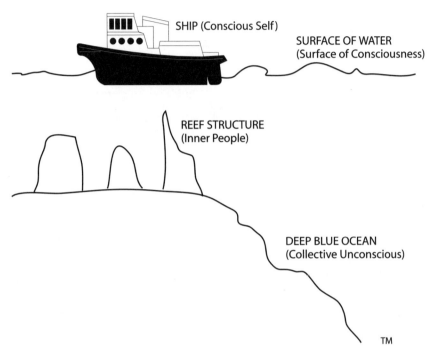

"As Figure 3 shows, the ship is analogous to the Conscious Self, the reef structure is analogous to the Inner People, and the deep blue ocean is analogous to the Collective Unconscious and Unconscious Self. All sea life emerges from the plankton in the deep blue ocean. The ocean has long been an archetypal symbol of the unconscious and dolphins, whales, and sharks have long been archetypal symbols of differing perspectives of that psychological reality."

Thomas then points over the side of the boat to the reef. "In the same way that the life of the reef and the ocean vitally affects our terrestrial existence, what goes on below the surface of consciousness vitally affects the life of the Conscious Self because the archetypal structure of the personality is the deepest foundation of all meaning."

Thomas turns the page on his flip chart to display a list of some of the archetypes. "I want you to take a few minutes and look over this list and try to get an *image* of each archetype in your mind, say each word silently, and feel any connection you might have with them, either with movies, or with books. Remember archetypes are metaphors that define the fundamental meaning of life, and the meaning behind all reality." Thomas backs away from the chart and leaves them to reflect upon the following archetypes:

ARCHETYPES MANIFESTED IN HUMANS AS INTRINSIC QUALITIES, ROLES, EXPERIENCES

persona	anima	mother
animus	father	hero
demon	shadow	seeker
rebirth	incest	destroyer
power	magician	divine child
trickster	warrior	lover
orphan	widow	wise old man
giant	birth	death
journey home	innocent	warrior
creator	fool	earth mother
virgin	prostitute	priest
inventor	wise old woman	friend

ARCHETYPES MANIFESTED AS MAN MADE OBJECTS, CONCEPTS, AND IDEAS

rings	weapons	the circle
quaternity	crystal	puns
riddles	parables	love
perfection	will	law
origin	faith	omniscience
plan	truth	

ARCHETYPES MANIFESTED AS NATURAL OBJECTS

trees	sun	moon
stars	wind	rivers
lakes	ocean	fire
mountains	streams	waterfalls
rocks	volcano	rain

ARCHETYPES MANIFESTED AS TERRESTRIAL ANIMALS

dog	cat	peacock
horse	squirrel	rabbit
monkey	bear	moose
eagle	buffalo	rat
snake	sheep	cock
boar	tiger	ox

ARCHETYPES MANIFESTED AS MARINE ANIMALS

dolphins	whales	sharks
manta rays	sea snakes	fish

ARCHETYPES MANIFESTED AS SENSE EXPERIENCES

red	gold	green
black	yellow	blue
brown	white	orange
purple	pink	bitter
sweet	sour	hot
cold	dry	wet
smooth	rough	loud
soft	pain	soothing

ARCHETYPES AS CLUSTERS OF BIOLOGICAL INSTINCTS

Sexual Procreation	Social Herd Instinct	Self Preservation

As Bethany scans the list of archetypes, at first she makes no inner connection to any of them. Suddenly, a powerful feeling comes over her when she comes to the word "rings" and she is reminded of the movie she had just seen, *Lord of the Rings*. She now realizes that the entire theme of the movie turns on the archetypal symbol of the search for the One Ring that could unify all the others.

After a few minutes, Thomas asks, "Anything jump out at you?"

James raises his hand, "I've always been fascinated by how Patton was profoundly convinced that he had been a warrior in a previous life. I'll bet he was driven by the archetype of the warrior."

Nikki quickly follows, "Harry Potter begins as the archetype of the orphan, and becomes the archetype of the hero."

"Yes," Thomas smiles at the group's enthusiasm. "This is a common archetypal theme that is also found in the *Star Wars* character, Luke Skywalker, and in the ancient myth of Oedipus Rex. Are there others that any of you connected to?"

Dan volunteers, "I've always seen the power of the archetype of the ocean in the movie *Titanic*."

Thomas chimes in, "Yes, that movie is filled with archetypal symbols. The ocean certainly is a symbol for the unconscious, and the story of the technical problem of finding the diamond that was supposedly still on the ship was interwoven with the metaphorical raising of Rose's memories about the ship. The sinking of the *Titanic* in the middle of the sea and the enormous loss of life, is a collective, archetypal example of the sinking and death of my own memory about my high school years, and the raising of those memories through my reconnecting with them at the reunion."

Thomas searches their faces for their level of comprehension, then asks, "What about the archetype of the journey home? The archetypal image of the hero is the theme woven throughout Homer's first book,

The Iliad, where Odysseus is busy conquering lands and defeating armies. *The Iliad* is a metaphor for the victories the Conscious Self achieves during the first half of life. Homer's second book, *The Odyssey*, picks up where *The Iliad* left off and tells the story of Odysseus' journey home to Ithaca aboard the ship Calypso in the hope of once again seeing his wife Penelope and son Telemachus. In stark contrast to the heroic achievements of *The Iliad*, in *The Odyssey* Odysseus loses his armies, his ship, and everything he had won in his former battles. *The Odyssey* is a metaphor for the psychological defeat of the totalitarian rule of the Conscious Self over consciousness. This is the first and necessary step to even beginning the archetypal process of the journey home. Carl Jung called this ancient process of the journey home Individuation. I call it the process of discovering who you are in the second half of life.

"Deep below the level of consciousness each person experiences themselves as strangely drawn to, or repulsed by, a subset of these archetypes, some more powerfully than others. An archetype is like a powerful magnetic field that attracts or repulses experiences, becoming a complex, or what I call one of the Inner People. No two Inner People will be exactly alike because individuals never have the exact same experiences in life, yet there are underlying themes to the character of the Inner People that the Enneagram describes. People also see evidence of archetypes as symbols in their dreams. Often the symbols are pressing the dreamer to address a collective, universal question in their own lives.

"The pattern of archetypal symbols in each of us defines the deepest foundation of all human meaning for us. In other words, as an archetype attracts life experiences, it becomes an individual answer to a collective question asked by all humanity. So the individual answer to the collective question about whether we are reborn after death is different depending on our life experiences, especially how we were raised. Archetypes *are* the meaning that has been assigned to nature and human creations both consciously and unconsciously by all people, in all cultures, in all times. They are the *a priori prototypes* of all things created by humans in all generations. They are the *ultimate foundation* of the paradigms of the world. They are the source from which the seemingly unfathomable depths of human emotion spring. The archetypes are the *source* of all inspiration and deep inner psychological energy. They are symbols that embody the ultimate existential questions in life."

"I recognize some of the archetypes on your flip chart," Nikki blurts out. "I once took a course in philosophy at NYU where we discussed Plato's notion of law, will, love, and truth as being *Platonic Ideas*. My professor said that such Platonic Ideas had become the foundation of all meaning in western civilization." Nikki looked at Thomas curiously. "Are you saying that Plato's Ideas are what you're calling archetypes?"

"That's exactly what I'm saying!" Thomas' face lit up with excitement. "The difference is that I view archetypes like law, will, love, and truth as biological-psychological *entities* that exist at the biological-psychological interface of the Collective Unconscious, not in some other *spiritual* world of Being or Essence like Plato claimed."

Some of the divers were confused by the discussion they were having, and Thomas picked up on this by the look on their faces, and resumed, "Nikki, let's discuss this privately after the session."

She nodded in agreement, and Thomas quickly said, "To return to what I was saying, the overall pattern of archetypal attraction that is present in you, along with your Conscious Self, Inner People, and Unconscious Self, defines the overall structure of your personality, as was shown in Figure 2. We experience the biological-psychological interface most clearly in the survival archetypes where we see biological processes when we look from the outside in, and psychological processes when we look from the inside out.

"The most important point to note is how much of the process happens outside the space of consciousness and the realm of the Conscious Self. The unfolding of the psychological map of the archetypes and the Inner People is a natural process that is *objective* to, and *independent* of, the Conscious Self. This is one of the most counterintuitive aspects of the model I'm presenting. Not only is the process objective to us, it is real because it makes a physical difference in the sense we defined before. We are actually drawn to and repulsed by archetypal forces that most people are not conscious of for most of their lives. These same forces are what define the path of our destiny.

"So with the vast majority of psychological activity in the personality happening far below the surface of consciousness, the question remains, 'Who *is* in charge of the personality?' The confusion and inner conflict that most people experience tells us that no one is—our inner life is a battle where one of the elements of the personality tries to gain total control at the expense of other elements.

"Some people find it disturbing to hear that the Conscious Self is only one of many complexes in the personality. Other people find comfort in this model because they have been acutely aware of the battle and have not known what to call it, or how to understand it from the perspective of being just one person.

"I'd like you to reflect on two things prior to the next session. First, do you feel threatened or comforted by the model of the personality presented? Second, look down into your emotions, then try to imagine them as the emotions of the Inner People who are looking back up at you in consciousness.

"I warned you that this session would be the most theoretical of the entire dive workshop, so I want to take some time to see if there are any comments or questions. Yes, Nikki."

"I don't get the switching perspective thing and the Inner People being objective from me, yet inside of me."

"Alright, let me give some other examples. When we got up this morning we all saw the sun rising over there," Thomas points east then west, "but now it is dropping in the sky, and tonight it'll set there in the west. Imagine that you could project yourself onto the sun and see the same thing from that perspective, what would change?"

Nikki says, "We would see that it is really the earth that's moving, not the sun."

"Right," says Thomas. "Our observations and beliefs even about common-sense things like the motion of the sun can be deceiving. Our observations about what we see in the sky are why people thought that the earth was the center of the solar system for so long. So in the case of the sun, the reliability of our explanation of what we see depends on our perspective, right? We see differently when we see from a distance. The same motions look different when we observe them from a different place or position, and we look different when we view ourselves from a different perspective."

Several people nod in agreement as things are becoming more clear.

"Let's try another example." Thomas walks to the boat railing, turns to face the divers, and says, "You selected a group of people to give you feedback on your 360-degree review. Reviewing their feedback is an attempt to get you to see yourself from a distance—from their point of view. But other people do not know your deepest thoughts, desires, and emotions, so imagine if you could project yourself into their bodies and observe yourself from their perspective. What would this add to the reliability of your definition of yourself?

"Finally, imagine you're standing in front of a mirror and the *you* that is looking into the mirror is the view of yourself that the Conscious Self has. What if the *you* that is staring back is the Unconscious Self and the Inner People who have the other side of the story of your life. What if you could project yourself into the mirror and view yourself from the perspective of the Inner People and the Unconscious Self? What would *that* perspective add to the reliability of your understanding of yourself?" Thomas walks back to the flip chart and says, "Does that help?"

Nikki is blown away, because the power of what Thomas has been trying to explain finally breaks into her conscious awareness with a blazing illumination that is like the noon sunlight.

"Are there other questions? If not, let's gear up and go diving."

Dan was pulling his wet suit out of the rinsing tank because he had forgotten to hang it up to dry after the last dive. There was nothing he hated more than trying to tug cold, wet neoprene over his warm body. As he continued dressing, the thought pressed into his mind that his Conscious Self was only one of many complexes in his personality and that the person he was today could have been otherwise. What hit him even more profoundly was the notion that the Inner People and the Unconscious Self provided him with compensatory feedback that gave him the other side of the story in his life. Dan's inner world had always been dominated by a deep, pervasive sense of inner judgment and incessant commentary on his life from what was like an army of inner critics. Formerly, he experienced these feelings as his, but now he could entertain the fact that this commentary came from the Inner People who were as much a part of who he was as the person who was sitting here on the deck of the boat. In a sense, the fact that the Inner People took over the facility periodically didn't relieve Dan of responsibility for his behavior, it rather intensified it because he was learning how to deal with these takeovers, like the kind that happened so long ago in the back of Cheryl's SUV.

Dan and the others were still dressing as Kirsten began the dive brief. "This will be a wall dive where the coral reef drops one thousand vertical feet straight down into an abyss, so watch your depth on this one. We'll do it as a one-way drift dive so we'll try to all get in the water together, drift along the wall with the current, then the tenders will come pick us up when we surface. It's important to limit your bottom time to no more than sixty minutes so we can all get picked up around the same time. If you're running low on air and have to come up sooner, just surface and one of the boats will pick you up."

Indonesia is famous for its capricious currents that can instantly rise to three or four knots, and then change directions, shift, or disappear without a moment's notice. These become manageable when you dive sites at a full-low or full-high tide, which was how the crew of the *Explorer* were doing it. In a sense, inner diving to explore the unconscious aspects of the personality was no different. You had to watch the enormous flow of power and psychological energy from the deep regions of the personality and only dive when the inner tides were just right. In a very real sense, the struggle between even an accomplished scuba diver and the ocean was metaphorically like the struggle between the Conscious Self and the unconscious.

The two boats full of divers had to time getting in the water just right because the current was screaming on the surface. As the divers from Mike's boat dropped down into the water, it became clear that the boat had drifted beyond their planned entry point, and they had entered the water just on top of the reef, which was only about thirty feet deep. Following Mike's lead, his divers began to frantically kick against a current that was at least two knots, in order to move a short distance across the reef-top and join Kirsten's group, who were already beginning to drop down along the wall. With a current this strong, the cloud of bubbles flowing from their regulators indicated that Dan and the other divers with Mike were huffing and puffing, breathing like race horses.

Finally they reached the wall and began to drop to their dive depth of about sixty feet. The current was moving at a good clip, but now they were drifting with it and could stop and catch their breath. With visibility that was this good, they could see Kirsten's group just up ahead.

The color of the coral on the wall was magnificent. The idea was for the divers to maintain a constant buoyancy and depth and let the current push them past the reef like a sight-seeing show. There must have been fifty kinds of soft coral-like trees waving in the current, and Gorgonian fans that were five feet high. As they were propelled past the wall by the two-knot current, Maggie could see the reef fish swimming against the current in order to stay in their current position.

About twelve minutes into the dive, the current slowed down, then instantly shifted directions—straight down. Thomas looked into the masks of his fellow divers and saw wide, unseeing eyes filled with terror as the current carried them to eighty, then one hundred feet, with no sign of slowing down. Mike signaled for everyone to get to the wall and just hang on. At about 130 feet their downward journey was stopped, only because they were pinned to the wall. The fear and stress only increased as they saw the fish on the reef swimming against the current, straight up toward the surface of the water.

Looking around at the other divers, Thomas saw that as they exhaled from their regulators their bubbles were going straight down into the bottomless abyss, and he could feel the pressure of the current trying to tug his regulator out of his mouth. Thomas had heard of inexperienced divers in Cozumel who had been caught in "down and out" currents. One couple, on their honeymoon, was carried down, then out to sea and never seen again. Thomas was now clinging to the wall for dear life as he also remembered a dive master in Bali who was carried to a depth of almost three hundred feet before he was able to get control of the situation and move back toward the surface.

Mike looked at his dive computer, and given their current level of nitrogen and their depth, he knew that if this current didn't quit soon, they would have to move hand-over-hand up the wall to get closer to the surface of the water. About sixteen minutes into the dive the current slowed, then stopped its downward motion. The divers looked at each other with an overwhelming sense of relief. Those last four minutes had seemed like an eternity. When Mike's group moved back up to their planned depth of about sixty feet they saw Kirsten's group, who had also been caught in this downward-flowing washing machine of water. Some divers were shook up to the point where they immediately surfaced and were picked up by one of the boats. For the divers who finished the dive, there was no current along the wall, so they meandered at a leisurely pace trying to catch their breath and make sense out of what had just happened. By the time they surfaced fifteen minutes later, the quiet, colorful world of the reef had put them at ease, but the terrifying experience of almost being swept into the depths of the sea would be indelibly inscribed in their hearts and minds.

Thomas was wondering what the divers would say when they got back onto the main boat. He had seen situations where people's lives were threatened underwater, but once on the surface they usually tried to smooth it over in a kind of macho way. Thomas was the last person into the tender. As it pushed its way across the water toward the mother ship, he heard Joel shouting over the whine of the twin 150s on the back of the boat, "Man, that current was screamin'." But the main focus of the discussion when they got back on the *Explorer* was how great the dive was and what they had seen. For most people, diving was this way. Once they were back on the surface of the water, they went back to the surface of psychological life. They talked about fish, the boat, or how tough the current was, but they rarely discussed the emotions they had experienced when they were under the water.

SESSION 3: HUMAN MOTIVATION—
WHY THE PERSONALITY IS AT WAR

The divers have finished a late lunch and are sitting around chatting as Thomas rings the bell for the group to assemble. People quickly grab a cold soda and wander over to their seats around the teaching table on the main deck of the boat. As he begins speaking, Thomas asks rhetorically, "Why is the personality bound in a civil war? The *central claim* of this session is that the deepest human motivation occurs at the biological-psychological interface where the elements of the personality are either *driven* by the basic fear of biological and psychological survival, or we are *motivated* by the basic trust that we will survive biologically and psychologically. The basic fear of psychological survival is why the elements of the personality war against each other. I will discuss that on two levels.

"The first level is perhaps the clearest example of human motivation because it occurs along the biological-psychological interface and is what I referred to in the last session as archetypal clusters of biological instincts: sexual, social, and self-preservation. Each of us has all three archetypal clusters that merge either with the archetypal core of the Conscious Self or the Inner People. The cluster that merges with the Conscious Self becomes more powerful than the other two because it gets so much reality time. Consequently, it becomes a primary motivation and driver for everyday behavior and attitudes toward life.

"We are less aware of the presence of the other two archetypal clusters because they merge with the Inner People and most of us are unconscious of their presence and effect on life. The sexual, social, and self-preservation archetypal clusters can be viewed biologically (outside-in) or psychologically (inside-out) much like a cloud can be viewed outside-in or inside out.

"When the sexual archetypal cluster merges with the Conscious

Self, we experience the biological side of the coin as an extra powerful attraction toward sexual reproduction that projects itself onto potential mates as a non-personal, collective act of passing on our genes, thus allowing the species to survive. We experience this on the psychological side of the coin as an extra powerful attraction that projects itself onto people who we long to *connect* with psychologically, with the goal of passing on our ideas and who we are through intense interpersonal interactions that are orgasmic in tone. When the social archetype merges with the Conscious Self, we experience the biological side of the coin as an extra powerful attraction that projects itself onto people or social situations that will give us strength and security in numbers—the herd instinct. We experience this on the psychological side of the coin as an extra powerful attraction that projects itself onto people and social interactions that bring us importance and enable us to find a secure place in the social order of things. When the self-preservation archetype merges with the Conscious Self, we experience the biological side of the coin as an extra powerful attraction that projects itself onto human comforts such as food, shelter, warmth, and the other things that help us survive. We experience this on the psychological side of the coin as an extra powerful attraction that projects itself onto creature comforts, making sure we get frequent potty breaks, snacks, and making sure the temperature of our surroundings is just right.

"Given the fact that we all have all three archetypes to one degree or another, which one do you most relate to and experience most strongly in your life?"

"I'm definitely a self-preservation type," Lindsey volunteers. "I always carry goodies with me when I'm traveling somewhere, I hate hard chairs like these, and in meetings I'm always battling with someone over the thermostat for the air conditioning."

"I'm a sexual type," says Dan. "I really like intense people, relationships and conversations. I'm pretty intense myself."

Nikki offers, "I relate to the social type. I care about where I fit in the scheme of things and I always make as many connections and relationships with people as I can. You never know when you're going to need them."

"What about the rest of you?" Thomas says as he sees some nodding heads. "Reflect on and try to identify which archetypal cluster describes your experience best, remembering that we have all three to one degree or another. You'll need that information during the first session tomorrow."

Thomas takes an unoccupied chair from around the teaching table, turns it around so the back is facing the group, and sits down to rest his feet. "Okay, the second level is the most fundamental and contains the basic drivers and motivators to which all other human motivations can be reduced. Abraham Maslow's *abundance-deficiency theory* is one of the most fundamental explanations of this level of human motivation. Maslow claims that psychologically healthy and fully functioning human beings are motivated out of *abundance*, while neurotic people are motivated out of a sense of *deficiency* or *basic need*.[13] Most psychological models about motivation are in some sense reducible to a kind of abundance-deficiency theory. I add an important component of dimensionality to this view by integrating it with Erick Erickson's notion of trust. For Erickson, children under the age of one-and-a-half have to solve the first of eight psychosocial dilemmas, the first of which is learning basic trust or mistrust. This includes trust of self and trust of the world. It appears to me that the basic element of abundance is a kind of trust in self and the world, a trust that our needs will be met, and this is an important element of viewing life through the lens of abundance.

"My claim is that at the biological-psychological interface, the most fundamental human motivation is a dialectic tension between the *Basic Fear of survival,* and a *basic need to trust that we will survive.* The Basic Fear of survival has both outer-world and inner-world dimensions because it involves trust in self (inner-world) and trust in the environment (outer-world). When we do not have what we need to survive biologically and psychologically, we are *driven* to meet these needs and we live life out of a deep feeling of deficiency, that is, 'the glass is half empty and needs to be filled.' This drive to survive is often accompanied by inappropriate and excessive levels of psychological energy that are experienced by both the person being driven and observers of their behavior. When our need to survive is met *reliably,* a sense of trust emerges that we will survive biologically and psychologically and this trust *motivates* us to live life from abundance, that is, 'the glass is half full and is adequate for my needs.' The excessive levels of psychological energy in the driven person are noticeably absent in the person who is motivated by abundance. But if circumstances change and our biological or psychological needs go unmet or become unreliable once again, trust in ourselves and the world begins to erode and we move back to being driven by the Basic Fear of biological and psychological survival.

"It's one thing to talk about the Basic Fear of psychological and biological survival, but it's quite another to experience it. Has anyone ever really experienced times in their life when they came face-to-face with the threat of biological or psychological death?"

James raises his hand. "One time I was heading down to southern Colorado to see a friend in a terrible snow storm and I thought I would take a short cut. It was a complete whiteout and I went off the road on the top of a steep mountain pass and ended up in a ditch. The snow was blowing so hard that when I got out of the car and tried to dig myself out, the wind just drifted the snow over the car faster than I could shovel. I got back into the car, but realized that if the snow drifted up over the car I would be snowed under just like I was in an avalanche. As I sat in the car wondering what to do, the reality that I might die out there and never see my family again came over me with a vengeance. Luckily a snowplow came by and pulled me out, but had he not seen me, I might not be here today. That was one time when I felt that basic level of survival fear."

"Any others?" Thomas queries. People look at each other, but no one says anything. Finally Thomas breaks the silence. "How about that last dive?" The tension in the air gets thick as Thomas probes into a topic that most divers don't care to discuss. Even the best divers experience this level of fear while diving, but few if any ever talk about it introspectively once they reach the surface of the water or get back on the boat.

"I'll tell you how I felt," Thomas volunteers. "I was terrified." He looks at Mike, who has six thousand logged dives under his weight belt. Mike says, "The only other time that has ever happened to me was once off the south coast of Nusa Peinida in Bali. It was a washing machine. Me and two other divers were pulled to over two hundred feet before we knew what hit us. It scared me then, and I felt the same way this time. We're lucky we got to the wall as quickly as we did."

Thomas continues, "Water weighs over seven pounds per gallon and we had tons of it moving over us at close to three knots. I looked into most of your facemasks and saw the fear in your eyes, but our ability to talk about the Basic Fear of survival became somehow inappropriate once we got back on the boat. Some divers will not process this fear and will forever be afraid of diving in strong currents. This fear is real in that it will affect where they will and won't dive and it drives them years after the initial experience. For other divers, surviving an experience like that will make them better divers. It builds their confidence so that they can handle these things and not panic. This is a Basic

Trust that you can handle problem situations like we just had. As for myself, on the last part of that dive, I felt a new sense of Basic Trust emerge in my diving abilities because I survived and learned from that experience.

"So it is in life. Some people are so powerfully driven and dominated by their Basic Fear of biological and psychological survival that avoiding this fear and anxiety becomes the solitary criterion for even the most pedestrian of life's decisions. For other people, they learn that life's problems can make them stronger, it increases their confidence in themselves and their ability to face the problems of life."

Bethany strongly relates to the concept of the Inner People providing the guidance needed to turn her Basic Fears about life into a Basic Trust in herself and the world. Her entire life is one cantankerous meeting with multiple people arguing their views, despite what she says. The constant conflict of the Inner People drowns out any sense of the calling, guidance, and teaching of the Unconscious Self. The only guidance she has ever known is external to her, for example, the preaching of ultra-fundamentalist ministers, and the fire and brimstone, letter-of-the-law interpretation of the Bible. Life has been confusing for Bethany precisely because she has never known who was in charge of her personality. Probably the only thing she does know for sure is that her life is dominated and motivated by fear and anxiety that goes to the core of her being. This makes her acutely aware of being driven by the Basic Fear of biological and psychological survival. Like Darwin's theory of survival, her life is one battle after the other as a weak human-animal who is trying to make it in a world where only the strong survive. In the wake of having just finished Session Two, one of the Inner People begins to press across the boundary of the fringe of her consciousness. When this person gets control of the facility, she becomes a lazy, lethargic person who wants to just relax, stay at home, and avoid the conflicts of life in the peace and comfort of a familiar setting. Bethany finds herself fighting to keep this Inner Person from rising further into her consciousness. She fears that if she stops pushing with the energy she manages to summon out of the fear of failure, she will never get moving again and will eventually slip into a kind of inner swamp of constant negligence and laziness.

Rick raises his hand, waits until Thomas recognizes him, and says, "All this talk about inner conflict makes me feel uncomfortable. My approach is to avoid conflict, and most times my problems just go away."

Thomas responds, "Well, my own experience is that those problems don't go away; they may get buried underground, or be driven out of conscious awareness, but they do not go away.

"You all know what serious conflict is between you and other people, but turn your eyes inward and imagine the inner life of the personality—the war between the Conscious Self, the Unconscious Self, and the Inner People. In the inner world, the Conscious Self is *driven* to maintain control of consciousness, investing enormous amounts of psychological energy in its defenses because it fears this struggle is a matter of life and death. In a sense it is, because the Conscious Self experiences its loss of control over consciousness as a kind of psychological death. In the same way, the Inner People only exist in a virtual state and are *driven* to take over the facility because their reality depends on them having control of the facility in order to make physical differences in the world. To remain in a virtual state is to not survive, so they are driven to take control of the facility from the same Basic Fear as the Conscious Self.

"On the other hand, when the Conscious Self repetitively submits to the Unconscious's perspective, experiences the psychological death that the loss of control of consciousness brings, *and survives,* a Basic Trust begins to emerge that it will continue to survive and be stronger because of the experience. The Conscious Self begins to be *motivated* by a sense of abundance where control of the facility can be shared with the other complexes of the human personality. In much the same way, when the Inner People see that the Conscious Self will *voluntarily* give them control of the facility when it is most important to them, a trust begins to emerge that they too will continue to survive by making real differences in life. As trust grows, the Inner People begin to be *motivated* by a sense of abundance where they can have appropriate control of the facility with the Conscious Self. The promise of the psychological survival of all the complexes in the personality builds an enormous *trust in self* that gives us a deep and abiding sense that the total personality is robust, balanced, and can survive the onslaughts of life. The Conscious Self, the Unconscious Self, and the Inner People come to the realization that no part of the personality will be killed off, banished, or sentenced to psychological isolation just to satisfy some other, more powerful, part of the personality."

The group is quiet. There are no questions because people just don't know what to say. Thomas's examples and the entire discussion have connected their Basic Fear and Basic Trust to their dive experience in a deep and profound way.

Thomas breaks the silence. "I want to add two points for you to reflect on. First, reconnect to the Basic Fear that you had on the last dive and try to connect it to other experiences that you have had in your life. Second, identify areas in your life that are driven by Basic Fear versus being motivated by Basic Trust. Are there any questions or comments? If not, let's get suited up while Kirsten gives us the dive brief on this site."

Following the dive brief, the group grabs their weight belts and begins loading into the two diving tenders.

∿∿∿∿

Diving gets people out of their heads and present in their bodies. One of the dive skills that does this more than any other is learning to relax and breath deeply. Above water, breathing falls below the surface of consciousness and most people breathe on automatic pilot. But underwater, the slow, relaxed, consciously performed in and out motion of a diver's breathing makes them conscious of their body in a powerful way. The bodily awareness of the diver's breathing, in combination with the fact that the sound of their air as bubbles is the only thing a diver hears underwater, is what makes diving so relaxing. Slow, constant, steady, conscious breathing is what connects the diver to their bodily existence in a powerful way.

The two groups of divers were within sight of each other in loosely organized clusters. Dan had dropped down to one hundred feet to get closer to a hammerhead shark that was lurking in the shadows out in the deep blue. After the shark shyly swam off, Dan looked up toward the surface of the water and saw the blurred fuzzy outline of the sun shining in the sky. He was floating motionless under ten stories of water. Then, about twenty feet up, there appeared a swarming school of about fifty barracuda circling in the water column above him. He was glad Cindy talked him into coming. He'd already learned a lot about himself, life, and diving, and the workshop had only just begun.

Following the last dive, the crew pulls up the anchor and the ship begins sailing east toward Komodo Island. The bell rings for dinner and when Maggie arrives on the main deck, she sits with Joel, James, Kirsten, and Mike. The steward pours her a glass of white Balinese wine and all the new friends she has made are sitting around what only three hours earlier was the teaching table. Now it is an elegant dining table complete with tablecloth and candles. Everyone is chatting about the day and basking in the cool night air as the ship moves forward through the water. During a lull in the conversation Maggie says to Mike, "I'm staying in Indonesia for another month after we get back from this trip and I want to travel around. What's the situation like up in Sulawesi for Americans traveling alone?"

"What *situation?*" Mike says in his typically cynical tone.

"Well," Maggie says, "I've been reading that there've been reports of terrorists operating in the south part of the island, and I was wondering what the latest scoop was before I decided if I wanted to go up there."

Mike and Kirsten both look at Maggie and then at each other with smug expressions. Mike turns back toward Maggie and finally says, "I know your government keeps stating publicly that there are terrorists operating here in Indonesia, but I say, 'Where are they?' Indonesia is a very small place where everybody always knows everybody's business. If there were terrorists operating here in Indonesia you would not be able to keep it a secret for one day."

Kirsten chimes in, "It's true, it's a very small, tight-knit place. I doubt there's anything going on up there that would be a problem if you went."

"Look," Mike says, barely concealing his amusement at what he views as Maggie's paranoia, "there are no terrorists operating in Indonesia, so just relax and go where you want."

Maggie would have normally taken Mike on in her competitive way. This time she decides to let it go. But what Mike could not have known, was that within four weeks, while Maggie was still in Indonesia, terrorist bombs would turn two tourist night clubs in the west coast resort of Kuta, Bali, into a blazing inferno, killing almost two hundred people, mostly Australians.

By now, everyone around the table has turned their attention toward the discussion between Mike and Maggie. As they look on in silence not knowing what to say, the mood at the table changes from a relaxed atmosphere of people sharing their experiences to one where you could have cut the psychological air with a knife. As a diversionary tactic that would take Mike and Maggie's political discussion out of the spotlight, Thomas says, "Kirsten, why don't you tell us about the shore excursion to Komodo Island to see the dragons tomorrow."

Relieved that he has steered the conversation in another direction, Kirsten says, "Sure. The park opens at eight o'clock tomorrow morning and we'll have both tenders ready to go at seven-forty-five so we can get there right at eight. The Komodo park ranger will give us a talk and show us around. It will take about an hour, then back to the boat for the first session. We'll just rotate the three sessions and dives from the point we get back to the *Explorer* and we should have time to fit everything in."

Day 2
DRAGONS ON THE BEACH AT KOMODO

Competency 2:

Follow the

Three Red Flags

THE DAY BEGINS

They have sailed all through the night and are anchored at the island of Padar off the east coast of Komodo Island and the Komodo National Park, home of the world's largest lizards. Dan is tired from a combination of yesterday's dives, the material presented, the movement of the boat on the overnight trip, and James's snoring. All this added up to a restless night of intermittent catnaps. Despite this, he is ready for the shore excursion to see the dragons.

After a fifteen-minute boat ride in the tenders they arrive at the island, and the first thing Dan encounters when he goes ashore is a group of hawkers trying to sell him local trinkets and offering to exchange U.S. dollars for Indonesian Rupiahs at a ridiculously low exchange rate. The central compound area of the park is a series of huts, elevated on three-foot poles. Even the tourists who know next to nothing about the Komodo dragon can see that this is to keep these creatures out of the buildings that make up the park headquarters. Two rangers greet the group, and after a brief overview of the island topography everyone wanders down a trail with one ranger in the front of the group, and one in the back.

Each ranger carries a stick that is about five feet long and has a *Y* at the top, not unlike the wooden part of a slingshot. The ranger who is leading stops, and there off in the woods toward the beach are five or six Komodo dragons lying in the shade. Komodo dragons grow to be about eight feet long and can weigh up to three hundred pounds. They are notorious predators and scavengers that will eat almost anything. They move in a slow, deliberate way, but the group has been assured that they can run down a person in no time, and if their razor sharp teeth don't kill you, the bacteria that grow in the rotting food that partially stays in their mouth will. After a few minutes, the ranger at the back of the group says, "Please, please!" Everyone turns to see him forcibly redirecting a dragon that has slipped out of the woods and is coming up behind. It becomes clear why the two rangers had assumed these positions.

~~~~~

Back on the boat, the bell rings and most people have already taken their seats around the teaching table and are chatting with Thomas. Joel and Rick are talking and looking out from inside the main cabin and it is sometime after Thomas has begun speaking that they finally wander out onto the main deck and take their seats. The primary reason they are there is to dive and both Rick and Joel are wondering if they have gotten into more than they had bargained for with all this introspective stuff.

SESSION 1: VIEWING OURSELVES FROM A DISTANCE

As Joel and Rick find their seats, Thomas is handing out a drawing. Each of the divers has two books in front of them that describe the personality typology that they took prior to coming to the dive workshop.[14] Some of the people are leafing through the books as Thomas begins. "As a reminder, the reason we hold the dive workshop here in

Indonesia is to totally remove you from the context of your life so you can see your life from a distance, like a spectator. Today, we want to learn how to build a second type of competency, namely the ability to follow the Unconscious Self to issues that need to be changed and to help us view them as spectators.

"To begin with, we will set the stage for viewing ourselves at a distance with two tools. The first tool is the personality typology called the Enneagram. Part of your preparation for this workshop was to take the RHETI which we sent you, forward the results to me, and then read and reflect on the description of your Enneagram type. Based on your scores and my model of the human personality, I have put all of your Enneagram type information up here on the flip chart." Thomas points to the following chart:

CONSCIOUS SELF	SHADOW SELF	INFERIOR SELF
Type 8 James	Immature Type 5	Immature Type 2
Type 9 Rick	Immature Type 6	Immature Type 3
Type 1 Dan	Immature Type 4	Immature Type 7
Type 2 Lindsey	Immature Type 8	Immature Type 4
Type 3 Maggie	Immature Type 9	Immature Type 6
Type 4 Thomas	Immature Type 2	Immature Type 1
Type 5 Joel	Immature Type 7	Immature Type 8
Type 6 Bethany	Immature Type 3	Immature Type 9
Type 7 Nikki	Immature Type 1	Immature Type 5

"Up until now, I have been talking about the conflict between the Conscious Self and the Inner People in generic terms. But the Enneagram type descriptions will describe the *actual characteristics* of the Inner People because each one is an Enneagram type. While all the Inner People long to take control of the facility to have some reality time, two of the Inner People are normally most troubling in our lives.

I call this ménage à trois combination of the two Inner People and the Conscious Self the *Triangle of Duplicity*. The sheet I just handed out describes this." Thomas waits for everyone to turn their focus to Figure 4.

Figure 4

THE TRIANGLE OF DUPLICITY

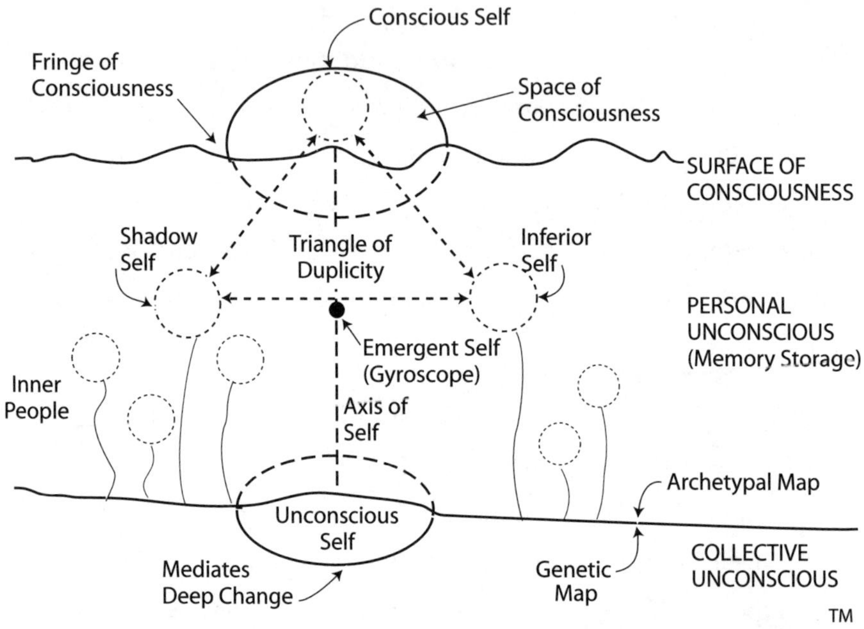

"Take Figure 4 and mark your Enneagram type number in the circle of the Conscious Self, then fill in the numbers for the Shadow Self and Inferior Self based on what I have up here on the flip chart. Then insert the other Enneagram numbers in one of the other circles to indicate the rest of the Inner People.

"Because the Shadow Self and the Inferior Self have been denied control of the facility for so long, they are like psychologically immature children who have been locked in a closet for the first part of their lives. The more completely they have been kept out of consciousness by the repressive powers of the Conscious Self, that is, your Enneagram type, the more psychologically immature they are. In practical terms, the lower their level of psychological maturity, the more inappropriately and contradictorily they act when they finally do get control of your facility.

"Let me give a brief description of how this Triangle of Duplicity affects us. First, the characteristics of your Enneagram type description concretely describe the characteristics of your Conscious Self. Your Enneagram type is primarily a typology of consciousness— that's why you recognize yourself when you read the description. If your type description were to describe unconscious attributes about you, you would not recognize them when you read them, and you would say, 'That's not me.' Although I will use the term Conscious Self, remember that your Enneagram type *is* a concrete description of the characteristics of your Conscious Self.

"The Shadow Self is one of the Inner People who exists below the fringe of consciousness, and regularly takes over the facility." Thomas steps out from under the tarp that covers the main deck and into the glaring sunlight on the deck of the boat. "Do you see my shadow and how it follows me? The Shadow Self is like that. It follows us around in our lives and when it takes over our facility, we behave in ways that are like an immature version of the Enneagram type of our Shadow Self. More importantly, when it takes over your facility, you experience the motivations, fears and emotions of the Shadow Self as your own. For all intents and purposes, you *are* that Shadow Self. But we normally only recognize a takeover after the fact, when the Conscious Self—your Enneagram type—has fought its way back into the space of consciousness. You can find the Enneagram type of your Shadow Self up here on the flip chart. For example, the Enneagram type that described Lindsey's Conscious Self is Type Two and the one that describes her Shadow Self is Type Eight. When you read the Enneagram description of your Shadow Self, you will probably recognize some of these characteristics in your life, although you may not be proud of them.

"The Inferior Self is one of the Inner people who exists in the deeper, darker regions of the unconscious, much further from even the fringe of consciousness. Its characteristics are so paradoxical to the Conscious Self that we can hardly even entertain the fact that this Inner Person exists within our personality. Because of its depth in the unconscious the Inferior Self has a kind of *cloaking device* like a Romulan space ship on Star Trek. The cloaking device makes the Inferior Self invisible so that the Conscious Self can look directly at the behaviors and emotions that it exhibits when it takes over the facility, but cannot see that this Inner Person has taken over the facility. But when you step back and view yourself from a distance in the spectator role, there will be distortions in the psychological energy field around the behaviors and emotions of the Inferior Self. When you examine the behavior and emotions you experience during a takeover with the descriptions of that Enneagram type in mind, you will begin to sense the presence and attributes of the Inferior Self more clearly. In the next session, after our first dive, I will describe these distortions in the psychological energy field as the Three Red Flags."

"Let me see if I have this straight, Thomas," says Bethany. "Since my Conscious Self is an Enneagram Type Six, my Shadow Self will be an Enneagram Type Three, and my Inferior Self is an Enneagram Type Nine. So in everyday life, when my Conscious Self has control of my facility, the write-up of the Enneagram Six should most closely describe my behavior."

"That's right," Thomas concurs.

Bethany continues, "But when the Shadow Self takes control of my facility, the Enneagram predicts that my behavior will be motivated by the description of an immature Three?"

"Yes," Thomas nods affirmatively, "and when your Inferior Self takes over your facility, the description of the immature Nine will most accurately describe and predict your behavior. That's why it's so problematic to be in a relationship with a person who is psychologically immature and who is subjected to the constant take-over strategies of the Inner People. You never know who you're dealing with, or who you're talking to."

Nikki says, "The approach to the Enneagram that I learned claimed that people were basically one Enneagram type, but could integrate or disintegrate to the other types along the lines of an inner flow."

"Nikki is correct," says Thomas, surveying the group. "Most Enneagram theorists claim that each person has all nine Enneagram types within them—that's why we get a score for all nine types on the RHETI. But these Enneagram theorists do not view the human personality as composed of numerous, independent personalities—what I call the Inner People, who can take over your facility and run your life. So the concept of an inner flow that integrates or disintegrates to the other Enneagram types becomes the way they explain the dynamic and ever-changing inner world of human experience. But this is another advanced topic that you and I should discuss after the session, Nikki."

"No problem," she agrees.

Thomas presses on, "Let's return to the notion that most people have little or no consciousness of the characteristics of the Inferior Self. When you read the Enneagram description of the immature version of your Inferior Self during the breakout time, you may have almost no consciousness of it, and find yourself saying, 'That doesn't sound like me.' But remember that being conscious of a complex in your personality is absolutely no indication of whether or not it actually exists and exerts causal power over you. The three Enneagram descriptions of the conflict within the Triangle of Duplicity will put a face on what we have experienced throughout the first half of life, and will continue to experience to some extent to in the second half of life.

"Also note that your own specific archetypal pattern will influence many aspects of your life. If a person is a Type One and has a powerful attraction, or repulsion, to the archetype of the mountains, they will probably do different things in life than a Type One who has a powerful attraction, or repulsion, to the archetype of the ocean. A person who is a Type Nine and has a powerful attraction, or repulsion, to the archetype of rebirth will probably be different than a Type Nine who is powerfully drawn to, or repulsed by, the archetype of the destroyer. Just as the three archetypal clusters of sexual, social, and self-preservation *color* how the Conscious Self appears, so do the rest of the archetypes.

"When we break out into working groups, I want you to read through the Enneagram descriptions of your Conscious Self, Shadow Self, and Inferior Self. Then, I want you to reflect on how well the descriptions actually describe the inner conflict you have experienced during your life."

Thomas begins handing out the results of the 360-degree review that he had tabulated and analyzed. "The second tool we will use to view ourselves from a distance is the results of your 360-degree review. This 360-degree review gives a well-rounded perspective of yourself because you received feedback from people in all the areas of your life: spouses, significant others, parents, children, friends, working associates, direct reports at work, and managers you work for. In the case of people who are presidents and CEOs, we asked for the perspective of members of the Board of Directors. As you know, some of the things we asked them about you were:

- How well do you listen?
- Do you value the views of others?

- Do you take feedback well, or do you get defensive?

- What are your blind spots?

- Are you trustworthy and do they trust you?

- Do you have a sense of personal responsibility, or do you blame others?

- Do you have control of your emotions (rage, anger, fear, sorrow)?

- Can you express your feelings appropriately?

- Do you respect their boundaries and physical and psychological space?

- What are your three biggest weaknesses and areas for improvement?

- What are your three biggest strengths, the ones you should capitalize on?

"As you review the tabulated results during the breakout time, remember to look for significant differences in the way you perceive yourself and the way others perceive you. Take about one hour to review the Enneagram type descriptions and the results of the 360. I will be here on the main deck during this time in case you have any questions."

Rick is like a person standing between two walls that are closing in on him, and he has both of his arms outstretched in the hope of fighting off the threat of being crushed between them. One wall is the pressure he is getting from his father-in-law about the business he had almost lost, the shame his wife felt over the situation, and the possibility that his life would once again be dismantled if he had to change jobs. The other wall that is pressing in on him is from the inner world of a mind that is spinning with anxiety and fear for his life. He spins scenario after scenario without any closure.

While he would never consciously admit to this, Rick has to lie and deceive people to smooth things over, and to get their approval. But one of the Inner People that Rick felt pressing into the fringe of his consciousness is someone who is tired of always being the doormat, the nice guy—the person who sucks it in and doesn't make waves. This Inner Person is tired of having to say yes to things, when he knows he has absolutely no intention of doing them, which in turn creates the image of incompetence that Rick has with so many people. This Inner Person has an enormous inner drive to succeed, be the center of attention, and will dominate the psychological space of life if it is allowed. But Rick quickly and ruthlessly drives this Inner Person out of his consciousness for fear that it might begin to pull the thread that will unravel the fabric of his nice guy, easy-going image.

Most people are blown away by how accurately the Enneagram descriptions have nailed them. But each person also takes the feedback from the 360-degree review differently. Some people got more positive feedback, others more negative, but no one is unaffected. No one can just stay on the surface. They are all pulled down into the deeper places in the psyche below the surface veneer that had typified the first day of the trip.

Joel finds the theoretical discussions of the structure of the personality and the biological-psychological interface of human motivation interesting and intellectually stimulating. But his attitude toward the dive workshop dramatically changes following the discussion of the Enneagram and 360-degree review. The Enneagram descriptions of the Triangle of Duplicity reveals one of the Inner People to be his Inferior Self, a person who longs to take over his facility and get revenge on people who have crossed Joel somewhere in his life. Behind the sterile intellectual exterior of Joel's Conscious Self is an Inferior Self who is a punitive, vindictive bully who intellectually and emotionally beats up on and abuses people who have wronged him. He is also annoyed about Thomas's reference to being led into an "inner wilderness." Ironically, this type of image of a barren wasteland is the precise Enneagram description of the inner landscape of his personality. His defense against the Enneagram description is to put on the persona of being skeptical and dismiss it as a waste of time.

But what really infuriates Joel is that the feedback that people gave him on the 360-degree review agrees with and validates the Enneagram description of the conflict in the Triangle of Duplicity. Other than the automatic skeptical response he uses to fight off any new information that threatens the image of his Conscious Self, he has no explanation for how this could have happened. Joel is furious about this feedback and tries to figure out who could have written these things. Rather than admit that he just cannot hide his true inner emotions and fears below his detached intellectual façade in a way that could actually fool people, he cannot wait to return to Los Alamos and debate the shades of gray with the people who gave him this feedback. Somehow he will find a way to get even with them.

Joel and Rick are sitting together talking. Joel has become more and more disgruntled about the whole diving workshop since yesterday, but this is really it. He and Rick feel that they have paid good money for this trip and too much of their time is being taken up by this workshop. They would rather do more dives each day. Joel finally decides to participate in a couple more sessions. But if things don't get better he'll ask Thomas to be excused from the workshop portion of the trip. Rick is getting downright uncomfortable himself and just wants to go home.

Thomas calls the group back together. "I'd like you to reflect on what was said about you in the Enneagram descriptions and the 360 and remember to entertain that what was said could be a valid perspective that you could learn and grow from—at least 10 percent of what you disagree with could be correct."

As Mike begins the dive brief, the divers start getting their gear on, but there is a quiet presence of introspection over the group, with the exception of Joel and Rick. Their reaction has not escaped Thomas's notice. He will just see where the situation goes with these two. The rest of the group had read the feedback they received from the people *they* had chosen, important spectators of their lives, and had taken note of what they said. Now each person will go down into the silent place of reflection where they cannot justify or rationalize themselves to others. The fish and the reef do not care.

~~~~~

Dan was shamed by the feedback he got. The differences between his positive sense about how he believed he interacted with people and what others thought of him were enormous. The written comments resounded with point after point about how critical, judging, hardhearted, and demanding he was in all walks of life. Dan had always thought that he was trying to help people by fixing things for them. But the written comments made it clear that people didn't want Dan's "help," but he gave it anyway. If they refused, he pounded them into capitulating with his misguided sense of self-righteousness.

One of his employees had made the comment, "He gets on your back and just won't leave you alone—he's a bulldog about everything." Dan wondered how his view of himself and the views of others could be so out of sync, as wave after wave of inner judgment began to break into his consciousness. His initial response was an enormous wall of defensiveness and rationalization as he said to himself, "If people would just get in line and do things right, most of these issues would go away."

The feedback from the 360-degree review was made even more

poignant by the fact that it was so thoroughly corroborated by the Enneagram description of his Triangle of Duplicity. All of his life it had taken an enormous amount of psychological energy for Dan to "manage" what he now knew was his Inferior Self—the Inner Person who cared nothing for the rules, being good, or doing what was right. On the few occasions when the Inferior Self had wrestled control of the facility away from Dan, he was instantly transformed into a glutton who just went and played, and did the things that were taboo when his Conscious Self had control of his life. When Dan finally grabbed himself by the scruff of the neck, snapped himself out of it, and got "back in his right mind," he had to make new resolutions to prevent these takeovers from happening. He forced himself to remember that life was about hard work, putting your shoulder to the grindstone, and just bearing up under life's heavy loads.

SESSION 2: FOLLOW THE THREE RED FLAGS

Thomas is standing at the railing staring over the ocean when Mike rings the bell for the group to reassemble. It's 11:00 A.M. and the steward sets a hearty snack on the teaching table because the group won't have lunch until about 1:45, after the next dive. Looking at the group that is now seated, but gazing slightly over their heads to the ocean beyond them, Thomas starts the session. "The vast majority of the ocean is deep blue sea and the majority of underwater topography even around an island like Komodo has sandy bottoms, and no coral reef. During our last dive workshop we decided to do some exploratory diving so I said, 'Let's just dive over there and see what we find.'"

Thomas points to a place on the other side of the bay from where the boat is moored. "There was nothing but sand. So how do you find the coral reef in such an enormous body of water when the total amount of coral reefs in the entire world represents a tiny fraction of the total area of the ocean? We find it by just exploring, but once we locate a good dive site, we tie a mooring ball that floats on the surface to a concrete block on the bottom somewhere near the dive site so we know how to find it every time we return.

"Finding coral reef in the vast ocean is not unlike finding issues in your life that will yield deep personal change. Of all the experiences you have had in your life, of all the conflicts you are aware of or that press into the fringe of consciousness, all the feedback you've gotten from others, where would you begin to identify the most important issues that need to be changed? How would you have any level of confidence that if you put your shoulder to the wheel and hammered through these issues, that this psychological work would really result in the kind of change we are talking about?"

James raises his hand and says, "I would look for themes in the comments of the 360-degree review and work on them."

Lindsey adds, "I would focus on the differences between how they viewed me and how I viewed myself."

Joel raises his hand and says cynically, "I am just going to keep on doing what I'm doing—after all, you said I was the final judge."

Several people are taken aback by Joel's cynicism. Maggie looks at Joel, makes a cynical face of her own, and says, "Maybe you should get into therapy to find yours!"

Thomas jumps in to regain control of the session. "James's comments are correct—we should look for themes in the feedback we get from others. Lindsey's comment about looking for differences is also correct. But we have to be careful about using the feedback of other people as the *only* source of information for identifying the crucial issues for us to work on. They could be projecting their own issues onto us so that their feedback is more about their own unconscious projections than our issues. If we only follow feedback that results from the projection of others, we will never resolve the problems we have, because the path we walk will not be based on psychological truth.

"Let's look closer at Maggie's suggestion. How many of you have been in any type of therapy or analysis?" About four people raise their hands. "Where did you start with them?"

Maggie speaks up, "Well, we normally began each session with my therapist asking me how my week was, and she used this question to find an area for us to begin discussing in the session."

Thomas nods, "That's good. Most therapists work in the realm of our Conscious Self with the goal of helping us get better adjusted to life. This is the approach of traditional self-help, using the therapist as a professional sounding board and guide to help interpret, or to learn to reinterpret our reactions to, and behavior in, life. But the necessary first step to deep change that we have been discussing is to abandon any hope of self-help because the root cause of our problems is the fragmentation and civil war between numerous complexes of the personality, most of which are not conscious.

"This is why Joel's comment about my own view, that we must be the final judge, raises such deep and penetrating questions about the material we are teaching, and the 360-degree review."

Joel is quite taken aback by this unexpected praise. But Thomas understands how cynicism plays out in workshops. If you fight it and let it get to you, it just gets stronger and can draw others into the contest. If you go with it and acknowledge any validity in the point, it dies under its own weight. Joel was visibly angry that Thomas did not take him on directly in front of everyone. This was the pattern of behavior that typified the way Joel disrupted things he no longer wanted to be involved with. The other people in the group were relieved at how well Thomas handled the situation.

"The *central claim* of this session," Thomas says, stepping toward the railing of the boat, "is that there are two shortcuts to finding the issues we need to work on, and they both involve following the Unconscious Self. The first short cut is to look for inappropriate levels of psychological energy. The second one is to look for evidence of the Three Red Flags.

"First, inappropriate levels of psychological energy mean that your emotional response to a situation *has you*, rather than you having an emotional response to the situation. It's when the level of affect that you display is entirely exaggerated and out of proportion to what was said or done. These enormous levels of psychological energy become stored around some issue or person that we have to deal with. People get consumed, taken over, grabbed by the scruff of their emotional necks by an issue that an hour earlier or later, even they would admit was not that big of a deal. When your emotions have you, they tweak you to the breaking point with the flip of a switch—when you're spring-loaded and toxic about some issue that you normally wouldn't care about, that's the telltale sign of inappropriate levels of psychological energy. These toxic releases can be overt and aggressive, or covert and passive-aggressive. They can be positive, like falling in love, or negative, like conflict between people. Whenever you detect emotional respons-es in yourself or others that are just not appropriate to the reality of what happened, stop dead in your tracks, get curious about what's going on, and mark this as an issue you need to work on.

"The second shortcut is to just follow the Three Red Flags." Thomas points over the side of the boat and asks, "Do you see that mooring ball over there? Excessive psychological energy and the Three Red Flags are like a mooring ball on the surface of the waters of con-sciousness that indicate an issue below the surface of our consciousness that we need to dive down and explore. Because the Unconscious Self comes from the deep blue waters of the Collective Unconscious, it knows where the issues that you need to work on are located in your psyche and it sets a mooring ball there—one of the Three Red Flags—so you can find it. They are:

- ♦ Unintended Consequences,
- ♦ Defense Mechanisms, and
- ♦ The Unconscious's Perspective.

"Like excessive psychological energy, when you see any one of these Three Red Flags, you should stop dead in your tracks and identify this issue as one of the mooring balls that leads to a productive place of exploration in the unconscious. Let me give you some of the highlights of all Three Red Fags.

"The first Red Flag is Unintended Consequences, which are disruptions of the intentions and actions of the Conscious Self. Look at Figure 5 in your handout. Let's say you are a manager and you have an employee named Jeff who really gets under your skin and causes you to experience excessive psychological energy in interactions with him. So your reaction is to ride him unmercifully." Thomas holds up his copy of Figure 5.

Figure 5

THE DISRUPTION OF THE CONSCIOUS SELF

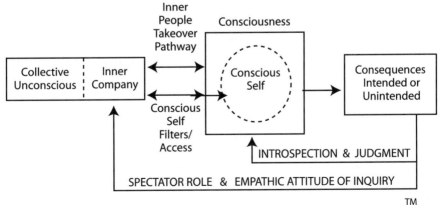

TM

153

"One morning on your way to the office," Thomas continues, "you decide that you really need to get off Jeff's back for both of your sakes. But fifteen minutes later, when you get to the office, you don't even have your coat off and you're on Jeff's back over a minor issue. As you can see in Figure 5, our tendency, when the goals and intentions of the Conscious Self are disrupted by an *Unintended* Consequence, is to go away from that situation, introspect about what we did, and judge ourselves for having failed. Judgment is normally the outcome of Unintended Consequences and judgment only leads to more and more judgment. The next day, during the pep-talk you give yourself on the way to work, you say, 'I need to *try harder* to get along with Jeff.' This time when you get to the office you last all of five minutes till you find Jeff chatting around the coffeepot rather than doing his work, and you light into him. Even though Jeff doesn't know you have been making and breaking these deals with yourself, you hammer yourself for once again failing. The next day, during your daily self-lecture on the way to the office you try a slightly different tack—the answer is that you need to *think positively* and focus on the things that Jeff does well. It's 10:00 A.M., you've made it through your first meeting with Jeff, and then he does something really lame, and you can't help but let him have it. In all these cases, one of the Inner People has taken over your facility. You—your Conscious Self—are almost helpless to stop it because of the surprise and power with which such instances break through the fringe of consciousness, throw you out of the president's office, grab the microphone of your facility's PA system, and start running your life the way they want. Unintended consequences provide powerful empirical evidence for the existence and activity of the Inner People, because if the Conscious Self really was the only complex in the human personality, disruptions of the behavior and emotional responses of the Conscious Self would not be possible."

Thomas puts both hands on the table and leans toward the group for emphasis. "When Unintended Consequences happen and people act really out of character with their Conscious Self, it is as if we are talking to *someone else*, but that someone else is in the same body as the person we thought we knew. We often try to make sense of these shifts in behavior or attitude by theorizing that the other person must be in a bad mood, upset about something, under pressure and stress, insecure, touchy, or a whole host of other attempts to make sense of and explain their behavior. But these theories are fabrications of the Conscious Self designed to preserve the illusion that it is the only complex in the human personality.

"While it is happening, we are often unaware of our dramatic shifts in attitude and behavior. Takeovers by the Inner People are often accompanied by enormous levels of psychological energy and intensity about some issue or experience that on reflection would hardly have bothered us at all. But while we are in the grip of a takeover by one of the Inner People, it's as if that is a life-and-death issue. Once one of the Inner People has control of the 'microphone' and the body, they can act in ways that they know will make the Conscious Self die of embarrassment, then they turn the facility back over to us and let us stand there and take the heat."

Thomas assumes a more relaxed stance. "It is only when the Conscious Self fights its way back into consciousness and drives the Inner People back down into the personal unconscious that we even notice that anything was wrong. So we normally become aware of a takeover after-the-fact when we've calmed down. In the wake of a takeover, the Conscious Self must assess the damage that has been done in this brief absence from consciousness. Using cues from the people or situations in the environment around them, the Conscious Self must cover up any evidence of the Inner People, so like the friends or colleagues who observe this happening to us, the Conscious Self fabricates theories to explain the takeover to himself. We experience this as the inner talk of the Conscious Self: 'I must be in a bad mood, or upset about something, or under pressure and stress, or insecure, or touchy.' Or we can come up with a whole host of other excuses to make sense of and explain the anomalous behavior. Likewise, the Inner People and Unconscious Self try to get their two cents in with the purpose of undermining these fabricated rationalizations. More times than not, the Conscious Self can successfully drive these opposing perspectives out of conscious awareness.

"But after this happens a few times, the Conscious Self becomes constantly vigilant and on its guard so that the Inner People do not take over the facility. This requires an enormous amount of time and psychological energy that could otherwise be used to live our lives and do productive things, but that is the price we have to pay for maintaining the myth that we are just one person."

Dan is finding it harder and harder to keep from staring at Maggie's incredible body that is turning bronze from the sun. As if on cue, one of Dan's Inner People starts pressing into his consciousness with a commentary on his behavior, "See how you want to stop staring at Maggie's body but you just can't!" Dan quickly snaps out of his reverie, as the inner voice continues, "That's precisely the kind of Unintended Consequence Thomas was talking about." This, in combination with his own defensiveness about the feedback he got on the 360-degree review, is quickly becoming empirical evidence that supports the principles he's learning—evidence that is not likely to go away.

Dan's incessant gawking at Maggie's body, and how quickly he turns away whenever she looks in his direction, has not escaped Maggie's notice. Dan's stares were beginning to bother her, and she wanted to give him a subtle message to *can it*. Maggie looks directly at

Dan, raises her hand, and says, "Thomas, how do you get a handle on these Unintended Consequences?" She adroitly turns toward Thomas and waits for his answer.

"Great question, Maggie." Thomas picks up the cue. "In order to move beyond such disruptions of the Conscious Self, we must abandon our attempts to try harder and think positively, and recognize that introspection and judgment that come from a unified sense of self only make matters worse. As shown in Figure 5, we must move into the spectator role and develop *an empathic attitude of inquiry, not judgment.* We must be open to the pressures that the Inner People exert on the fringe of consciousness and enter into an open dialogue of empathic inquiry with them about what it is that they really want, without any tone of judgment. The reason they normally act so psychologically and socially immature when they finally do get control of the facility is because locking them out of consciousness prevents them from becoming a mature, contributing part of our personality. Their absence from consciousness produces a kind of truncated lack of dimensionality in our overall personality."

Maggie and Dan are making direct eye contact across the teaching table, and although no words are exchanged, Maggie's question and Thomas's response tell Dan that he has been caught in the act. Maggie breaks off eye contact as Thomas steps toward his flip chart and says, "The second Red Flag we need to watch out for is Defense Mechanisms. Defense Mechanisms are problematic because they are designed to purposely distort and obfuscate our knowledge about ourselves and other people and prevent us from knowing the psychological "truth" of a situation. We experience the presence of Defense Mechanisms around two foci of confusion. We can't quite figure out:

- ◆ What we are feeling, and
- ◆ Whether the source of the problem is in others, or ourselves.

"Defense Mechanisms belong to the Conscious Self who refuses to allow us to be consciously aware of aspects of our inner and outer world, and prevents us from clearly understanding the emotions we experience. In order to maintain the illusion that it is the only complex in the human personality, the Conscious Self distorts and obfuscates our emotions. Consequently, when we ask, 'What is it I am feeling right now? Why am I so bound up emotionally? Why do I have so much inner tension about this issue? Why am I so upset about this issue?,' we honestly don't know because the Conscious Self either totally prevents us from becoming conscious of the true reason or relegates the emotions to the fringe of consciousness. The net result of this gate-keeping process is it robs us of our freedom to experience ourselves and life the way they really are by denying us access to our own emotional life, which is actually the emotional life of the Inner People that we experience as our own. We are not only prevented from experiencing the emotions of the Inner People, because this would challenge the solo existence of the Conscious Self, we are also prevented from hearing the calling of the Unconscious Self to discover who we are in the second half of life.

"Luckily, the Inner People refuse to be shut out of consciousness, so they project their unacceptable emotions, impulses, and thoughts onto people and the external world in such a way that we are almost totally unaware that this is happening, and the Conscious Self attributes these projections to other people. We really believe the problem is *out there* with other people in the world, and the Conscious Self uses its Defense Mechanisms to produce experiential evidence to maintain this illusion so it does not have to recognize this as the work of the Inner People. That is why when we become bound in enormous levels of psychological energy, the Defense Mechanisms are designed to confuse our ability to answer questions like, 'Are the causes of this interaction in me? Are the causes of this interaction in others? Are the causes of this interaction in collective phenomena? Are the causes of this interaction some combination of factors? Which combination is causing the problem and why?'

"The Inner People continue to project themselves out onto the objective world in the hope of forcing the Conscious Self to channel more and more of its psychological energy into keeping its defenses up. The strategy of the Inner People is to eventually defeat the Conscious Self at its own defensive game. The Inner People project themselves onto people and situations in the external world in the hope of causing more and more interpersonal conflict. This forces the Conscious Self to channel more and more psychological energy to protect itself against external challenges, and weakens the inner lines of defense along the boundary of the fringe of consciousness, making it easier for the Inner People to take over your facility."

"I've heard people talk about projection as if it was something they consciously did—you know, 'I'm projecting my own issues onto you,'" Lindsey speaks up. "But that's not what I hear you saying."

"That's right, Lindsey." Thomas starts pacing as he continues, "The unconscious Inner People project themselves out onto the world, and most times the Conscious Self sees the problem as happening 'out there,' not as an inner struggle. In fact, the Conscious Self fights to keep the projection out there in the world. But once we understand the nature of this inner conflict, we can help to isolate, and hopefully eliminate this type of battle, with a principle that helps to identify the root causes of problems of which we are unconscious.

"I call it the *Projection Principle*. In the *negative* dimension of the Projection Principle, we always hate what we secretly are. In other words, any time we are bound up in excessive levels of emotional energy, where some issue has us, rather than us having an issue, it almost always points to some projection on our part. In the *positive* dimension of the Projection Principle, we also always love, and are powerfully drawn to, what we secretly are. The excess psychological energy that is linked to our projections becomes a psychological mooring ball that hovers over an inner dive site that lies deep below the surface of consciousness. We then explore that inner dive site using an empathic attitude of inquiry, not judgment. We ask questions like, 'Why do I have so much positive or negative energy around this issue? What is it in the other person that has some metaphorical or real counterpart within me?' Answers to this empathic line of inquiry do not come from the Conscious Self, but emerge on the fringe of consciousness without any conscious effort on our part to 'answer' them.

"Now, for a point of contrast, I want to return to my earlier comments about self-help books and therapists who help people work through issues that have to do with the Conscious Self. It's not that the Conscious Self won't pursue change. On the contrary, the Conscious Self will submit to almost any type of change imaginable, *except* the kind of deep personal change we are discussing here. This is because the first step to deep change is for the Conscious Self to lower its Defense Mechanisms and admit that *it is not* the only complex in the personality. As such, the Conscious Self's problem-solving strategies are unlikely to identify *acknowledging its own limitations* as one of the solutions to the problem of obtaining deep change. The Conscious Self *actively opposes and undermines* any evidence of the Inner People and the Unconscious Self."

Maggie says, "I have actually experienced what you call the Projection Principle with a person at work. I had this toxic relationship with one of my direct reports named Rachel. We struggled with interpersonal conflict for years even when we were peers, but when I was promoted to department director, long-standing problems between us intensified. I hired a professional coach named Luke, and during my coaching sessions I would describe all the things that got under my skin about Rachel. Luke told me the same type of thing you just said about hating who I was, and said I should look for my issues where I had lots of psychological energy.

"One of the things that just *infuriated* me was when Rachel would undermine my authority in meetings by taking cheap shots at me, like pointing out mistakes and stupid things that I did when we were still working together as peers. She did this just to embarrass me. I talked with her about it privately and told her to leave our past problems out of present situations. She would agree, but then she would do it again. One day over lunch, I was describing how I had really shut Rachel down in a meeting by reminding her of something stupid *she* used to do when we worked together, and Luke said to me, 'Maggie, that sounds like a cheap shot.' I must have had a quizzical look on my face, and there was a deafening silence. Finally, I said, 'What do you mean?' Luke waited a few seconds as the tension in the air grew and again asked me, 'Who does that sound like? Who takes cheap shots at people in meetings by bringing up the past?' Finally, I said, 'Rachel does.' 'That's right,' Luke said.

"It was amazing—once I recognized it as a projection, the energy that I had toward Rachel was halved almost instantly. I felt like I was focusing on the real issue, and most of my inappropriate energy about her was gone. My relationship with Rachel improved dramatically, and I began to see other relationships where what you call the Projection Principle was operating and work through some of that stuff. This one principle has helped me enormously."

"Yes, that's exactly what I'm talking about, Maggie," Thomas says, slapping the table with his palm, "We always hate what we secretly are. It is a brutal standard to impose on yourself, but I have almost never seen it fail to be true. Even when you have absolutely no idea what the issue within you is that's projecting itself, write it in your log-book with a star by it, and put it on the back burner. Sometime, someplace in the future, the Unconscious Self will guide you into a sit-uation where you will be able to see the psychological reality of the situation."

Thomas has wandered over to the other side of the teaching table where Maggie is sitting during this exchange of ideas. He turns and begins to walk back toward his flip chart. "Let's move on to the third Red Flag, which is the Unconscious's Perspective. We experience this in two ways:

- Ideas, insights, thoughts, emotions, and motivations that pop into your head from the fringe of consciousness, and

- Dreams that penetrate into consciousness.

"The experience of the Unconscious's Perspective along the fringe of consciousness is a common one that most people have all the time. Extend your arm as far as you can so your hand is just slightly less than 180 degrees to the side of your head. Move your hand back and forth in and out of your field of vision." Thomas waits for them to per-form this motion. "That's called the fringe of your vision. The fringe of consciousness is similar in that ideas, insights, thoughts, emotions, moti-vations, and even guidance on critical issues in our lives just seem to pop into our heads 'out of nowhere.' By now, you understand that this nowhere is somewhere, that the place these revelations come from is the unconscious realm of the Inner People and the archetypes.

"It is important to write down experiences that appear on the fringe of consciousness for a number of reasons. First, it is a way of acknowledging the contribution of the Inner People in the human per-sonality. The Inner People provide a unique perspective on life and powerfully augment the problem-solving capabilities of the Conscious Self by giving us the other side of the story, and through creative solutions. When we act on their suggestions, the Inner People become real in a powerful way, and this lessens the conflict in the Triangle of Duplicity because the Inner People come to trust that you will give them charge of the facility voluntarily. Eventually they will no longer feel that they have to take over the facility by brute force.

"The second reason it is important to record experiences that appear on the fringe of consciousness is because this is where we often sense the calling, guiding and teaching presence of the Unconscious Self. Writing these experiences down codifies them and lets the Unconscious Self know we are listening. Reviewing what we have written in times of confusion or turmoil will often reveal patterns and potential paths forward around problems that we would have otherwise missed.

"The other way we experience the Unconscious's Perspective is through dreams that penetrate into consciousness. Although a detailed treatment on dreams is beyond the scope of the dive workshop, I want to talk about three aspects of dreams:

◆ Type,
◆ Purpose, and
◆ Interpretation.

"In terms of the *type* of dreams," Thomas brushes the sweat from his brow, "everyone dreams every night and the vast majority of dreams never penetrate to even the fringe of consciousness. The function of most nightly dreams is to process the conscious and unconscious data of myriad everyday experiences, worries, and interactions of life into the memory structures of the personal unconscious. Some of these dreams have sufficient psychological energy to penetrate into consciousness, meaning we remember them when we awake in the middle of the night, or in the morning. Most times these dreams are *personal* in nature in that they are the commentary of the Inner People and the Unconscious Self on our conscious life, that is, our relationships with friends, family, workers, activities we participate in, plans we make, and various other elements of conscious waking life. Since the Conscious Self filters out the elements of our experience that it views as a threat to its psychological survival, the censored aspects of our waking experiences become part of the data set of the Inner People— the other side of the story that we talked about earlier.

"Carl Jung proposed a second type of dream that he believed contained archetypal symbols that were spontaneously produced by the Collective Unconscious, independent of the intentions of the Conscious Self. Archetypal symbols exist at the biological-psychological interface in the Collective Unconscious of all people, at all times, and in all societies. Primitive cultures called this second type of dream a *big dream* and viewed these apparitions of the night as having collective tribal significance. In ancient Greek and Roman culture, such dreams were required to be reported to the Areopagus or to the Senate.[15] Today, many people encounter the archetypal symbols in their dreams when they are facing particularly important psychological situations, and at decisive moments or periods over the course of a lifetime. Jung proposed five periods.

- Childhood: three to six years old,
- Puberty: fourteen to sixteen years old,
- Young Adulthood: twenty to twenty-five years old,
- Middle Age: thirty-five to forty years old, and
- Prior to Death."

Thomas pauses and closes his eyes for a second as if to recall one of his own dreams. "Okay, let's discuss the *purpose* of dreams which is almost always *compensatory*. Dreams that contain *personal symbols* give us compensatory feedback on our everyday activities in life and relationships from the perspective of the Unconscious Self and the Inner People. These commentaries on the Conscious Self are often brutal, so it is important to view dream images symbolically—again, with an empathic attitude of inquiry, not judgment. So if you dream that you are lying in bed side-by-side with your ex-husband who you absolutely hate, or a manager who you despise for having no values, this may be how the Unconscious Self visually communicates the *Projection Principle*. So what you hate about the person in the dream is somehow true about you, but you are unconscious of this aspect of yourself.

"Dreams that contain *archetypal symbols* give us a compensatory window into the foundation of all human meaning. The Unconscious Self uses archetypal symbols to reveal our destiny, and the individual path that we must walk in answer to the collective, existential questions of humanity. It reveals the direction and path of discovering who we really are. So whatever the dream images are, we should approach them symbolically with an empathic attitude of inquiry, not judgment.

"Finally," Thomas stares intently at the group, "the *interpretation* of dreams is not straightforward, but it is a skill and a symbolic way of thinking that can be learned. The Unconscious Self almost always speaks in the language of stories, puzzles, riddles, parables, and puns, not the concrete sequential forms that so dominate the vast majority of our waking life. Consequently, the symbols and images in dreams should almost never be taken literally. Rather they should be viewed as a metaphorical and symbolic commentary on consciousness from the perspective of the Inner People and the Unconscious Self. The best way to approach dream symbols is with an empathic attitude of inquiry that tries to tease the symbolic meaning out of the symbols by asking questions that don't necessarily have direct answers. For example, it's common to have the setting of a dream be in a house you live in, or once lived in. The symbol of a house often represents your psychological life because your house is where you keep your material possessions—the *stuff* that gives people so much of their conscious identity. The empathic attitude of inquiry would ask questions such as, 'Why would the Unconscious Self pick this particular setting for a dream at this particular time in my life?'

"In many cases, the meanings that your unconscious associates with personal symbols are an *accidental* consequence of your life experiences. For example, a man who loves a woman and is planning to marry her takes her on a trip to Chicago for the purpose of proposing, and during the trip, the woman breaks up with him. From that point on, hearing the city's name will probably be associated with pain, sorrow, or loss for the man. Had she accepted his proposal, he would probably have associated Chicago with happiness and joy. In such cases, the meaning associated with the given symbol, Chicago, can have very different associations and meanings from person to person. This is why so few symbols have any kind of fixed meaning.

"Unlike the other aspects of the Three Red Flags, dreams not only point to the existence of the Unconscious Self and the Inner People, they actually put *a face* on the Inner People and relate them to personal and collective experiences that we have in life. You should also have an empathic attitude of inquiry when you've had a dream about a person of a known Enneagram type because the Unconscious Self will also try to give you commentary on the unconscious from this perspective."

Lindsey's hand goes up, "Once I had a dream about a person at the office who I absolutely hated from the first time I met her. I could hardly stand to be in the same room with her and I was forced to work with her quite closely. In the dream, I walked up to the house I lived in as a child, opened the door, walked into the living room, and there this person was. I said to her, 'What are you doing here, this is my house? Get out!' 'No,' she barked back at me, 'this is my house. You get out!' We went back and forth in the dream for who knows how long, and I woke up in a panic. Somehow I intuitively knew exactly what you just said, that there was a part of me that was like her. The next day when I went to the office, the enormous level of psychological energy and defensiveness that I had toward her was almost gone. I see now that this was what you're calling the Projection Principle. I was hating in her what I secretly saw within myself."

Thomas says, "Yes, Lindsey's dream points to the hidden life and objectivity of the Inner People. Whenever there are inordinate amounts of psychological energy in our relationships, there's almost always someone else 'in our psychological house.' Lindsey, did you write that dream down when you had it?"

"No," she replies, "it has stayed in my memory since that time because of how powerful it was."

"I would write it down even now," Thomas urged. "Use the logbook you got with the workshop and write down everything you can remember about it, even images and fragments of the dream. Whether or not you have any idea what the meaning is, write it down. Even if the scenes and symbols seem moronic, stupid, and of no value, write it down. Logging our dreams raises the material into consciousness in a way that simply trying to remember them does not. More importantly, writing a dream down honors the Unconscious Self and the Inner People and gives them the message that you are open to the Unconscious's Perspective and their commentary on your Conscious Self."

"But I just can't seem to pry myself out of my warm bed in the middle of the night to write them down," Nikki says.

"Try keeping a pen and paper on your nightstand so you don't have to get out of bed," Thomas offers. "Or, what I do is talk my dreams into a hand-held tape recorder, then play it back and write them down in the morning."

James chimes in, "But then I'd wake up my wife."

"Look," says Thomas, throwing his arms wide apart, "what is your alternative? If you wake up in the night or in the morning and are depressed, sad, lonely, terrified, or are captivated by some disturbing effect, if you have the dream symbols recorded in your journal, you will have some visual sense of what caused the feelings. If you don't write the dream down, you will be haunted by the effect of troubling emotions throughout the day, and have no hope of knowing what the cause of these emotions is."

Thomas relaxes his stance. "I now want you to think about two things. First, reflect on instances in your life where you saw the Three Red Flags. Second, reflect on the Unconscious's Perspective that comes through fringe consciousness or dreams you recall.

"Are there any questions? If not, let's go diving."

Kirsten steps up to give the dive brief. "The first fifteen minutes or so of this dive will be a shark feed. We will maneuver the tenders on top of our entry point, which will be a sandy channel about eighty feet deep, through which the current is screamin'. Mike will get into the water first at the north end of the channel with a milk crate filled with barracuda heads, rotten fish, and spoiled food from the trip, and will drift to the point of the shark feed. We'll drop in at the north end and drift with the current till we see Mike on the bottom. When you see Mike, stop, grab hold of a rock, or set your reef hook into a non-living part of the reef and just wait there."

Mike cuts in, "I will wait till you are all in place, then I will take the top of the milk crate and let some of the fish heads out. You will see two-foot, dog-toothed tuna begin to swarm around the milk crate and as more and more fish heads come out, the tuna will go into a wild feeding frenzy. Then the sharks will show up and all hell will break loose. When the fish in the milk crate are gone, the tuna and sharks will leave just as fast as they came. Then we'll unhook and drift to the end of the channel where the water slows down around some beautiful coral heads. That's where we'll spend the rest of the dive. Make sure that you watch your bottom time and nitrogen levels for the first part of the dive, and if you have to break away from the group before we finish, just drift to the end of the channel and we'll meet you there. Any questions?"

Dan was hooked to an enormous rock at the bottom of the channel just twenty feet from where Mike had the milk crate. It happened just like he'd said, but it was faster and more furious in real-time. The dog-toothed tuna were in a frenzy instantly, and then came the sharks, swimming full force into the swarm of tuna fighting over an enormous barracuda head. The shark grabbed it effortlessly, almost as if the tuna just let go, knowing the pecking order of the food chain. Bam! Dan turned around just in time to see a shark swim past him, having just smacked him in the arm with its powerful tail. Dan's heart was beating at a furious pace. Shark after shark continued to barge their way into the crowds of tuna and swim away with their catch.

Finally, the milk crate was empty and James, Dan, Thomas, and Maggie unhooked from the places they were perched at, and drifted toward the end of the channel. Maggie loved the dramatic and competitive feel of the reef where prey was pitted against predator in a struggle for survival, Darwin right before her eyes. But nothing revealed this competitive struggle more than the shark feed, because there she witnessed how the predator at the top of the food chain who has ruled the ocean for over a million years does business.

Lindsey was relaxing as she hovered over an unimaginable array of colors that were alive and teeming with life. With the deep penetrating questions that Thomas was forcing the group to face, Lindsey was beginning to feel like she was melting down emotionally. Last night when she'd returned to her cabin, she found herself quietly weeping in the darkness and hoping that she wouldn't awaken Kirsten, who was sharing the cabin with her. She had no idea where these emotions came from or the depths to which they reached. The first session today only turned up the heat. The written comments on the 360-degree review—about her thinly disguised inner conflict between wanting to be a loyal resource to Mario and wanting to run the company from behind the scenes—cut to the bone. She actually felt a sense of shame about the observation on how she flattered people and was a brown-noser. But as painful as it was, she could not deny these things. They were her dark side, the part of her that she rarely faced for fear of what she might find. While these parts of her seemed to be perfectly visible to others, it became clear that she had enormous blind spots in these areas.

What was equally penetrating was the Enneagram description of her conflict in the Triangle of Duplicity. On the last dive, one of the Inner People pushed her way into the fringe of consciousness and Lindsey got a powerful glimpse into one of the most problematic of the Inner People, the Inferior Self. This Inner Person was like a spoiled, pouting, spiteful little brat who kept score of who got what in life, and became green with envy when people did not respond to her manipulation, or she didn't get what she thought she deserved. The Conscious Self that Lindsey had always identified with tried to present herself as a kind, helpful, self-sacrificing person who wanted to do nothing but serve others, but when the Inferior Self took charge of Lindsey's facility, the people she interacted with were puzzled and sometimes angered by her duplicity. What was most shameful and left her feeling most vulnerable about what she was learning through the dive workshop was that she could not keep these darker elements of herself hidden from the world like she once thought she could.

SESSION 3: THE CONSCIOUSNESS MATRIX

It is three o'clock and the sun has already begun to sink from its zenith in the sky. Mike rings the bell that signals the start of the final session for the day. Thomas is turning a page of the flip chart as he begins, "The Consciousness Matrix is a kind of summation of much of what we have covered thus far, but in a single diagram." He points to Figure 6 on his flip chart.

Figure 6

THE CONSCIOUSNESS MATRIX

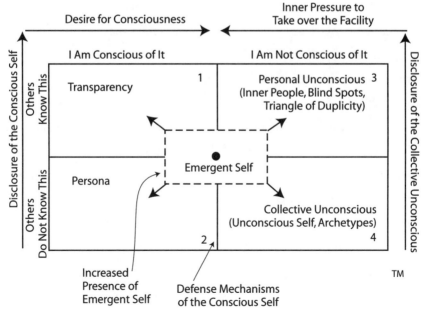

"Let's just take a few minutes to review the basics of Figure 6, then I'd like you to break up into groups of two or three and try to relate the *central claims* of the sessions we've covered thus far to the four quadrants of the Consciousness Matrix. Notice how the Defense Mechanisms of the Conscious Self form a barrier between the right-hand and left-hand quadrants. The natural path by which consciousness occurs is from Quadrant 4 to 3, and then to 2, then 1. In other words, the deepest archetypal elements in the Collective Unconscious disclose themselves through the Inner People, which then migrate to the hidden aspects of the Persona and then to the Transparency quadrant.

"As a result of this path of consciousness, part of the information in the Persona quadrant is information that I know about myself, but choose either to disclose, or not disclose to other people. Another element is partial information I know about myself in terms of an unintended consequence, but do not know how to disclose even if I wanted to, because these issues exist on the fringe of consciousness and I don't know how to formulate them into cohesive linguistic descriptions. In the absence of clear knowledge about myself in these areas, I fabricate theories to explain my own behavior to myself and to others, whether or not I ever choose to disclose them to other people.

"We only have so much psychological energy in the human personality and the Persona quadrant can become spring-loaded and toxic by the everyday interactions of life. Pressure can build and toxicity levels rise to the point where it requires an enormous amount of psychological energy to keep the contents of the Persona quadrant from bursting into the quadrant of Transparency because the differential pressure between the two quadrants becomes so large. When we are in the presence of a person who has large levels of differential pressure between Quadrants 1 and 2, we often feel that we have to walk on eggshells and watch out for land mines. If we were to question this person about our impressions, they would be aware of what we were talking about, even though they might still be unwilling to disclose this to us.

"When Quadrant 3 becomes spring-loaded and toxic, this can result in an enormous differential pressure that we will be unaware of, but other people may sense it in us, or we may see it revealed through instances of the Three Red Flags. Spring-loading and toxification of Quadrant 3 is much more serious than Quadrant 2 because of our unconsciousness of the problem. A spring-loaded and toxic Quadrant 3 is what we normally call truly neurotic behavior.

"The most serious scenario is when Quadrant 4 is spring-loaded or toxic with the raw, primitive, archetypal energy of the Collective Unconscious. When these non-personal, archetypal forces break in on the other three quadrants like a raging river, this results in an enormous differential pressure between one or more of the other quadrants, and can actually fragment the psyche and cause serious neurosis or psychosis. This differential pressure then rises up into the Personal Unconscious quadrant and eventually to the Persona quadrant in the form of dreams that penetrate into consciousness. The life-long process of discovering who we are is the process of the movement of psychological material through the four quadrants and the releasing of psychic energy to do the productive work of the personality. It is also the process of *waste management* where we process the toxicity that builds up in the quadrants through the everyday interactions of life and experiences. During the discussion time, write your insights and observations about the Consciousness Matrix in your logbook so you can keep them for future reference. Okay, let's break up into our discussion groups for the remainder of the session."

Dan teams up with James and Lindsey. Lindsey volunteers to lead the discussion and asks, "Who wants to start?" Dan, with a serious look on his face, says, "I will. My mind has been wandering to my relationship with my wife Susan and my daughter Carol. These have been some of the biggest battles of my life over the years. I have always assumed that having a good relationship was just a matter of finding the right thing to do, then doing it. But the Consciousness Matrix shows me that it's really the totality of *all* our personalities that are brought to bear in the arguments that I get into with Susan and Carol. I'm beginning to see that it's really the disconnection between the parts of our personalities in the Transparency and Persona quadrants, and the negative interaction between my Inner People and their Inner People that are crucial factors in our disagreements. No wonder my relationships with them have been so difficult and complicated." James and Lindsey nod in agreement as Lindsey continues the discussion by sharing her experiences.

When the hour of group discussion is completed, Thomas calls the divers together around the teaching table and asks, "Are there any insights that you want to share based on the exercise? If not, let's go diving."

Everyone in the group has plenty on their minds, but they want to get into the water so they can reflect in the peace and tranquility of the underwater world.

~~~~~

James, Lindsey, Maggie, and Dan had been talking about trying to see some "big stuff." This dive was a one-way drift drive along another magnificent wall of coral and sea life, but these four agreed that forty-five minutes into the dive they would move away from the wall and allow the current to take them out into the deep blue.

Somehow Lindsey got separated from James, Maggie, and Dan just before the forty-five-minute point in the dive, so she stayed with the main group, as these three blue water explorers moved away from the wall and let the current begin to take them out to sea. Almost instantly the wall was no longer visible, and they were floating buoyantly at sixty feet over an ocean floor that was a thousand feet below them.

Blue water diving can be disorienting because there is no solid point of reference and it's easy to just drop into the blue abyss without noticing it, so all three of them had their eyes glued to their dive computers so they could monitor their depth. Five minutes into this part of the dive, they looked down into the deep blue, then at each other, and finally at their dive computers. Nothing yet.

Out of the corner of her eye, Maggie spotted an enormous creature rising straight from the ocean bottom, then she spotted a second and a third—manta rays; there were four of them altogether. These gentle giants can grow to have wingspans of up to eighteen feet. Related to the shark family a million years ago, they evolved into placid creatures who open their three-foot-diameter mouths and scoop up billions of microscopic plankton, their main source of sustenance. Over and over again these huge animals swam up and within five feet of Maggie and her two friends. It was almost like they were playing a game of hide-n-seek. They would disappear into the blue depths only to reemerge and loop underneath them again.

The divers' air was low and they had already logged a sixty-four-minute bottom time, so they signaled to each other that they had to head up to the surface. When they hit the surface, the driver in the tender heard them before he even saw them as Dan yanked his regulator out of his mouth and screamed as if he were a baseball fan rooting for his home team in the World Series.

The bell to signal dinnertime rings at 7:05 P.M., and about half the group is already sitting around the teaching table, which has been set for dinner, but has also taken on a special function for this group of divers.

The teaching table has become a kind of "sacred space" within which to share with each other and learn. The steward announces the menu for the evening as Mike and Kirsten begin pouring wine and bringing the first course. As so often happens in these kinds of settings, there are several conversations happening simultaneously and usually people will drift from topic to topic until some point of discussion has enough critical mass to draw everyone's interest to a table-wide discussion. This night, that doesn't happen. The mini conversations cover a wide spectrum of topics from how you go about picking a dive destination when the magazines make them all look like the best one in the world, to having children and the positive effect they have on your life. The talk is light, unpretentious, and flows seamlessly. Thomas takes this as a sign that people are really relaxed, enjoying the diving and enjoying themselves.

Day 3
THE COOL WATERS OF THE INDIAN OCEAN

Competency 3:

Wait for the Synthesis

of Opposites

THE DAY BEGINS

Sometime in the early hours after midnight, the *Explorer* begins sailing to Nusa Kode on the southeast side of Komodo Island, where they will get to explore one of the most famous dive sites in Indonesia, Cannibal Rock. Dan is rocketed from sleep by a dream. In the dream, he was lying in bed, side-by-side next to his dead father whom he hated with a passion. In the darkness of the cabin, and in a semi-conscious state, it seems to take forever for Dan to piece together where he is. The rolling motion of the boat through the water makes something click in his mind and he realizes that he is on the *Explorer*, doing the dive workshop. Dan lies in his bunk paralyzed by fear and a sense of shame about the fact that although he avoided it his entire life, he has actually become like his father, Jake, in more ways than he has been willing to admit.

The motion of the boat stops in the water, and Dan hears the crew dropping the anchor. Even though it is only 5:45 A.M. he smells coffee brewing, and when he climbs out of the lower bunk to get dressed, to his surprise James is already up and gone. He climbs the stairs to the main cabin, grabs some coffee and sits down with James and Lindsey who are chatting quietly. "Do you mind if I join you?"

They look at each other, then at him, and after a slight pause James says, "Sure, we're talking about a dream I had last night."

Dan says, "I had one too—or maybe it was a nightmare."

James looks at Lindsey and says, "I was asking Lindsey how she dealt with the dream she shared with us in class yesterday, and I had just started telling her mine. My dream contained a single image where I saw myself lying on a table like the wooden teaching table on the main deck, and I was having open-heart surgery. The feeling I had when I woke up was deep to the marrow of the bone, but I'm not sure what that feeling was. It kind of felt like it led to an inner wound that was deep within me, and somehow in the dream, through the surgery I was being healed."

Lindsey asks, "What was yours, Dan?"

Dan is touched by her interest. "Well, I dreamed I was lying in bed next to my father who died last year. I was actually relieved when he died and felt a sense of freedom because he was always so verbally abusive and I hated him so much. I've spent a lifetime trying to avoid even the slightest appearance of being like him, but I have a sense that this dream is saying I haven't succeeded."

"I can't tell you how much I hated that woman in the office," Lindsey shakes her head. "And when I saw her in the dream symbol of my house, I realized that I was really like her in more ways than I was willing to admit. Back then I didn't know to call it Thomas's Projection Principle, but I really did hate in her, what I secretly knew about myself."

James breaks in, "It was weird, I woke up in the middle of the night, turned on my bunk light, wrote the dream in my logbook, then went back to sleep. When I woke up early this morning, I still had the feelings associated with the dream, but I had totally forgotten what the dream content was about until I reread what I wrote in my logbook."

"Yeah," Dan says, "I need to write mine down before I forget it. Now I know what Thomas meant by how these sessions would stir up the unconscious. I'm going to talk with him about the dream privately."

Most people are feeling the physical pressure of doing three tanks a day, and they begin straggling in to breakfast in the main cabin as the usual Mozart plays softly in the background.

Breakfasts on the boat are custom: the steward takes your order for eggs, French toast, or any other breakfast fare you want, and there is always a buffet of fresh fruits, cereals, coffee, and every kind of tea you can imagine. The dive workshop is not the place to come to lose weight.

The sun is shining brightly and even before the bell rings at 8:00 A.M., people have migrated to the main deck where Thomas is busily writing at his flip chart. Rick and Joel sit together as usual, talking in a whisper. James, Lindsey, and Dan sit together because they are beginning to feel a strong sense of bonding to each other. Somehow, they are all on the same journey, but for different reasons. They are all answering the calling to deep personal change.

SESSION 1: THE INNER WILDERNESS

"Today we will cover material for the Third Competency," says Thomas, "which is waiting for the synthesis of opposites from the spectator role. The *central claim* of this session is that the defeat of the Conscious Self as the totalitarian ruler of consciousness is the first necessary step to enabling the Unconscious Self to organize, harmonize, and unify the fragmented and warring complexes of the personality into an integrated whole.

"The evidence of the Three Red Flags is used by the Unconscious Self to bludgeon the Conscious Self into the recognition that it is not alone in the human personality, with the goal of humbling it. It's not unlike punching holes in the boat of the Conscious Self so it takes an enormous amount of energy to psychologically bail out the boat of consciousness just to stay afloat in the storms of life.

"The pounding that the Conscious Self takes from life, the Unconscious Self, and the Inner People leads the Conscious Self into a kind of inner wilderness where we realize that we no longer have the answers to the questions of life." Thomas gestures with his hands, "I mean questions like, 'Who am I? How should I interact with the world? How should I live now in light of it all? What does the future hold for me? Why can't I stop doing this? Why can't I start doing that? Why can't I be more aware? Why can't I be less aware?'

"Being in the inner wilderness is like being caught between our past self (the Conscious Self) and the self we have yet to become (the Emergent Self). The prospect of being trapped in the inner wilderness is simply demoralizing for the Conscious Self who has always been in charge of the facility, and determined the course of our lives. The inner wilderness is like a holding cell of total uncertainty where we are forced to turn our face into the inner desert of our lives, that dry, barren, lifeless wasteland that so many of us run from and never come to terms with. As we wander in this desert, even the tracks we make are blown over by the hot, driving inner winds of our spirit, leaving us without reference and without the ability to know where we are or where we need to go.

"It's hard to explain how much psychological energy it takes to keep the helplessness of the Conscious Self in consciousness. Just try it." Thomas challenges them. "Think back to the most emotionally charged situation you've been in during the last six months, one in which inappropriate levels of energy *had you* and you said or did something you regretted. Or hold a dream image in your mind like Lindsey's dream where the unconscious gives you the feedback that what you hate in someone else, is a part of who you secretly are."

Dan thinks about how hard it is to hold the dream image of him and his dad in his mind and to entertain the idea that they were two sides of the same coin. The thought of it raises every psychological defense he has, but Dan is trying to move into the spectator role where he can entertain the validity of this commentary on his Conscious Self that rises from the Unconscious's Perspective. The dream pits self against self and reveals the core problem of the inner civil war. But if one of Dan's Inner People *is* like his father, and if this Inner Person has been getting control of the facility all these years, the dive workshop is showing him the way out of this unconscious, self-defeating way of living. He doesn't have to identify with the Inner Person that is like Jake. He can move into the spectator role and allow the Unconscious Self to mediate the battle for control of the facility—the battle for consciousness.

Thomas continues, "The function of the Unconscious Self in the human personality has *always* been to organize, harmonize, and unify all complexes in the personality, but the fragmentation and warring of the Inner People prevents this from the earliest days of our lives. As I just said, the first step to beginning the process that was meant to start so long ago is to defeat the Conscious Self, but as we have seen, this is no easy task. The Conscious Self must be forced to abandon its self-appointed totalitarian control over consciousness and its defenses must be worn down to the point of collapse. Most importantly, the Conscious Self must be defeated, but it must not be destroyed because *all* the complexes have a role to play in a personality that actually becomes whole for the very first time in life.

"The Conscious Self experiences its loss of power over consciousness as a kind of impending psychological death, and fears this fate like James feared being stranded in that snowstorm, or some of us feared the deadly force of the current two days ago. As I mentioned yesterday, when we are identified with the Conscious Self, we experience its emotions as our own. That means we experience the defeat of the Conscious Self as *our* defeat. We experience its loss of control over life as *our* lost control, and we experience its psychological death to be *ours*. When we are identified with the Conscious Self we experience the trauma of being stranded in the inner wilderness. But leading us to this place of death, and forcing us to stop identifying with the Conscious Self is the stated goal of the Unconscious Self. Otherwise, our personality that was destined to be made whole will remain fragmented by the on-going inner civil war."

Joel and Rick glance at each other, then Joel turns toward Thomas, raises his hand, and barks, "This sounds like masochism!" He turns toward Rick, then looks at the group in disbelief, and continues, "What kind of *normal* person would subject themselves to this kind of psychological torture?"

The air is charged with tension as Thomas calmly responds, "Well, Joel, it's not unlike preparing for a marathon or any other kind of physical exercise, like diving."

Joel leans over and talks to Rick, paying no attention to Thomas. "Initially," Thomas continues, turning his attention to the others, "when we get our bodies in shape, this causes physical pain. But when we stay with it, the pain subsides and we are stronger because of it. Psychological growth is no different. In fact, what is most important is that we must not try to squirm out of the enormous inner pressure and psychological pain that we must endure in the inner wilderness. The only way that the power of deep, profound, sustainable change can be unleashed in our lives is if we stay in the process till it's completed. If we run, escape, or try to resist the process in any way, we will only have to face it again, and next time we may be less prepared or able to endure it.

"Rather than trying to avoid or escape the inner wilderness, we come to see it as a necessary part of the process of answering the calling to discover who we really are. It becomes a partnership where we learn that the Unconscious Self actually wants to *collaborate* with the Conscious Self in the process of deep change. What the Unconscious Self asks of us is that we help it intensify the change process by purposely allowing instances of the Three Red Flags into consciousness, and holding them there for as long as we can. In other words, instances of Unintended Consequences, Defense Mechanisms, insights from the fringe of consciousness, and dream images that the Conscious Self fought out of consciousness with the Basic Fear of its own survival, must be *held* in consciousness, with an empathic attitude of inquiry, not judgment."

James raises his hand and asks, "Thomas, is Lindsey's dream about Rachel an example of how this process works?"

"Absolutely!" Thomas responds. "In the inner wilderness, the Conscious Self must face the fact that it cannot produce deep change— it must experience this type of psychological death in order to live again in the wholeness of the personality."

The introspective nature of the material along with the enormous focus on deep change has caused the psychological pressure to build in Nikki. But Thomas's discussion of the inner wilderness has struck a chord in her that she does not fully understand and she decides to ask for clarification of his points.

Nikki raises her hand, and begins speaking with an uncharacteristically slow and reflective tone in her voice. "Somehow the inner landscape of my psychological life *is* like an inner wilderness. Even at this moment as I'm speaking, I feel connected to a barren, dry, windblown, and lifeless place that I have been running from my whole life. I have tried to escape the reality of this inner wilderness and place of emptiness by filling it with things, people, experiences, in a way that now, in retrospect, seems gluttonous. Your comments about the defeat of the Conscious Self, Thomas, have forced this into my conscious awareness. By staying in motion, all I created was an illusion that I had escaped this inner place of death to the Conscious Self. What I am now so keenly aware of is that I have confused my planning, frenetic escapism, and the illusion they created, for the reality of my life." As Nikki continues, a sensation of relief permeates her facial expression and tone of voice. "Being caught in the inner wilderness means that I am inescapably bound within the *existential now*—the place between the self I have always been, and the self I have yet to become. I have always chosen to flee from the pain and inner anguish of that place, and all I have succeeded in doing is to put off facing what could not go away. I think it's time for me to stop running."

Thomas and the others are humbled by her openness, depth of self-understanding, and vulnerability. What they cannot know is that because she has planned to attend the dive workshop for the last six months, Todd's feedback is included in the results even though he has been out of her life for some time. Although the respondents on the 360 are anonymous, Todd's open and brutally honest tone is not difficult for Nikki to identify. She is also acutely aware of the reality of the Inner People as described in the Enneagram description of her type. Being forced into an introspective focus by the dive workshop has lowered her natural defenses against the inner world, and the Inferior Self has been pressing heavily on the door of consciousness. This Inner Person is stingy, miserly, and retentive, and when it takes over the facility, Nikki will withhold herself, time, money, communication, and any other resource in life that she feels will be taken from her. This paradoxical Inner Person will hide from life and the engagement with life as if she is profoundly detached from people and a world that she doesn't feel she belongs in. The workshop is forcing Nikki to face the very things she has run from her entire life, and to take stock of that which exists under the persona of a happy, sunny person who just moves on when life gets tough.

Thomas looks at Nikki, who seems withdrawn into the inner world, and softly says to the group, "I have added two things for you to reflect on. First, given what you wrote on the 3x5 about what brought you here, ask yourself, 'Am I in the inner wilderness?' Second, 'Has the workshop helped me to define a path forward?' Are there any questions?"

Rick is caught on the horns of his own dilemma. He recognizes much of the Enneagram descriptions of the inner conflict in the Triangle of Duplicity, but the closer this new inner consciousness hits the mark with penetrating accuracy, the more Rick feels himself digging in his heels to avoid facing it and having to actually do something about it. He is face-to-face with the actual possibility of deep personal change. He can no longer say that he doesn't know how, or he doesn't understand. Having lied half-consciously his entire life, this will be a lie that he *knows* he is telling. More importantly, Rick is visibly stressed by the feedback that his father-in-law, wife, and employees gave him in the 360-degree review. The veneer of his nice guy image is barely masking his simmering rage at what they said. Every bit of evidence that was presented in the Enneagram and the 360 is calling him to take action. But Rick is so deeply mired in an inner swamp of psychic quicksand that the prospect of real change threatens to take him deeper if he tries to act on the truth of what he knows about himself. It is the dive workshop that is bringing all this to the surface. He figures that he and Joel will just drop out and spend the remainder of their time diving some of the finest coral reefs in the world. When he gets back to Chicago, things will work themselves out like they always do when he just goes with the flow.

Joel has had enough! He has a deep need to be left alone in his own little world and the workshop has gotten far too intrusive into his psychological space for his liking. Deep inside, Joel knows that the new information he is getting in the dive workshop is pressuring him to start making changes that are in his best interest. But his compulsive tendency to "stiff-arm" even legitimate change has kicked into high gear. Joel wants to change enough to keep his marriage together, but the dive workshop is much more than he'd bargained for. If he has to he will endure another divorce rather than seriously disrupt his research with all this change "stuff."

Thomas's question is still ringing in the air as Joel and Rick get up and stalk off to the bow where they commiserate about how sick they are of all this talk of inner wildernesses, deaths to self, and the *Projection Principle*. It's a waste of good diving time in a beautiful place that they probably will never get back to. This is the trip of a lifetime and they aren't going to waste it sitting in some classroom, even if it is on the deck of this ship. They decide they will wait till after the dive then let loose on Thomas and tell him that they want out of the dive workshop.

When Thomas sees Joel and Rick get up and leave the session early, he knows that the situation with these two is coming to a head, but he tries to hide his concern for the sake of the rest of the group. In his typical way he says, "Okay then, if there're no questions, let's go diving."

During the dive brief, Mike had warned them that the water temperature down here in the southern part of Komodo was cooler, maybe as low as sixty-eight degrees compared to the eighty-three-degree water they had been diving in. The temperature drop was because of the cold water currents from the Indian Ocean that fed the channels between the islands. Mike and Kirsten both put on their seven mil wetsuits. Most of the others in the group put three mil shorties over the top of their wet-suits and added a few more pounds to their weight belts. Dan just put a three mil hood on because you lose 80 percent of the heat of your body through your head. When they rolled off the side of the tenders and hit the water they could instantly feel that they were diving in a different temperature than they had been.

Dan liked diving with a hood. Not only did it keep him warmer, but it softened the sound of his bubbles. As if the world down under wasn't quiet enough, the hood helped to hush the only sound that could be heard. The steady, slow breathing of an experienced diver not only gets you out of your head and into the body, it also makes the normally rigid boundary between the unconscious and conscious much more permeable. Dan was purposely holding the dream image of him and his father in consciousness as Thomas had suggested. As he stayed present to the dream image, he felt inner forces trying to pull him back into the conflict in the Triangle of Duplicity as some of the Inner People pounded him mercilessly with judgment and condemnation. He stepped outside the conflict in the Triangle of Duplicity, then was pulled back in, then forcibly he extracted himself from the conflict and moved back into the spectator role. This was exhausting psychological work, but as he moved in and out of the inner conflict, it seemed to become easier, almost like the way you build endurance at exercising or weightlifting.

Joel and Rick corner Thomas after the dive and Joel jumps all over him. "Look, Thomas, Rick and I are tired of these work sessions. They are a waste of valuable time that we could be spending diving. We want out of the dive workshop now!"

Rick just stands there and says nothing, but he appears to agree with what Joel is saying.

Thomas asks, "But what's the problem? You seemed to be getting into the material yesterday, so what's happened between then and now?"

Joel says, "The Enneagram is a waste of my time. Besides, I came here to see what Indonesia's diving was all about, not to sit in a classroom all day." Rick is still silent, and now takes a step away from Joel.

Thomas replies, "But the Web site and the material you got when you signed up clearly said that the sessions and dive time were equally split. I don't get it." Then, trying to probe at the real problem, Thomas asks, "Joel, what's really wrong?" Thomas looks at Rick, and then at Joel and says, "How do you explain the fact that the tabulated results and written comments of your 360 and the descriptions in the Enneagram Type Five and Type Nine match so well?"

Joel loses his temper and bellows, "It's more complicated than a simple mapping!" With this outburst, Rick takes another step away from Joel, and still says nothing.

Thomas can see that confronting Joel will only make matters worse, so, as a concession, Thomas offers, "Look, Joel, I want you to enjoy yourself on the trip and if you want to do more dives, I'm sure I can arrange that."

When Joel sees how accommodating Thomas is being, he begins to cool off.

"So long as it doesn't conflict with the dives the workshop is doing," Thomas offers, "you and Rick can take shorter surface intervals and while we are in sessions, I'll have the boys load you up in the tender and take you out to one of the nearby dive sites. You can even do a night dive after dinner if you want and get up to five dives a day. But I just want to remind you not to push your nitrogen limits too far with the shorter surface intervals. If you get bent out here, it's a thirty-four-hour boat ride back to Bali, which is the only decompression chamber for a thousand miles."

"Fine," says Joel. "We can live with that, right, Rick?" Rick nods in half-hearted agreement.

"How do you want me to handle telling the group?" Thomas asks. "Either you can tell them or I can, but they have to be told directly, and up-front."

"Why don't you just tell them at the start of the next session that Rick and I are dropping out to get more diving in, and they can come to us if they want the details," says Joel, now wishing he hadn't lost control of his anger with Thomas.

"Sounds good, that's what I'll do."

After Thomas walks away, Joel looks at Rick in disgust and says, "Thanks for backing me up, buddy. Did your mouth quit working or what?"

"No," says Rick, blushing slightly. "I just couldn't think of anything to say. I don't like that kind of conflict."

"Really?" says Joel, as he shakes his head and walks away.

SESSION 2: THE INNER DIALECTIC OF DEEP PERSONAL CHANGE

The steward has just finished bringing multiple plates of food to the teaching table as a snack when the 11:00 A.M. bell rings to start the next session. Joel is noticeably missing, but Rick takes his normal seat at the teaching table. Thomas is only half surprised to see Rick show up. He explains to the group that Joel has decided to get more diving in and leaves it at that.

The group had seen Rick and Joel conspiring and overheard Joel yelling at Thomas after the last dive, and they are actually relieved about Joel dropping out. But they are surprised that Rick chose to stay on. His body language makes it clear that Rick really doesn't want to be here—

it is as if he's trying to make himself invisible to the group, and in all the discussions he's checked out somewhere up in his head. But when push comes to shove, Rick just can't deal with the conflict of not returning to the group. Saying one thing, then doing another, is part and parcel of Rick's style. Joel couldn't care less. He prefers diving alone anyway. The duplicity between Rick's outer behavior and his true feelings only puts more pressure on him, because Joel's departure serves to increase the positive psychological energy of the group and help them focus more on the teaching, the very thing that makes Rick's skin crawl. With each passing minute, Rick just becomes more and more invisible, and the rest of the divers quickly forget he is even there.

Thomas begins, "The *central claim* of this session is that the Unconscious Self must mediate the conflict between the Conscious Self, the Triangle of Duplicity, and the other Inner People as we look on as spectators. All we can do is to wait for a synthesis of the opposing views that is mediated by the Unconscious Self. The inner civil war has been between the Conscious Self and the Inner People. During the first half of life, the Unconscious Self has been trying to carry out its organizing, harmonizing, and unifying functions, *to no avail*. When we hold to a unified view of our personality, we experience all of these conflicting voices as our own because they all reside within our body.

"But when we stop identifying with the various complexes of the personality, we realize that these issues belong to them, not us. We must come to see our childhood identification with the Conscious Self as an illusion. We must increasingly allow the presence and influence of the Emergent Self to become *real* in the sense that it makes a physical difference in our personality and in how we live our life."

Thomas turns the flipchart pages back to Figure 4, and asks rhetorically, "These are the complexes of the personality we have been describing, but where are you in this drawing?"

Figure 4
THE TRIANGLE OF DUPLICITY

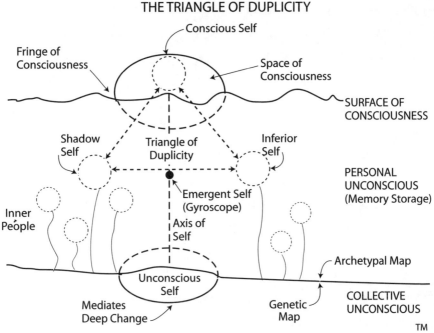

Their eyes are intently focused on the diagram, and one by one Thomas sees their curious faces turn to look at him. "You are looking at the diagram as a *spectator*. From this perspective, you see the warring complexes of the personality as objective and independent from you. Do you see what I'm talking about?"

Some of the people in the group look confused. He waits a few seconds, and then says, "Another way to describe the objectivity of the spectator role is that you become like Dickens's character, Scrooge, watching his life pass before him and seeing himself the way others have always seen him."

The name Scrooge triggers something in Dan's mind because he has always felt a shameful kinship with this Dickens character. Dan says, "So, in the story, when Scrooge was standing there with one of the spirits, *looking at himself* during his childhood, watching that person dance and fall in love, and watching himself deny Bob Cratchit and his son

Tiny Tim any human kindness, this 'watching of self' is what you're calling the spectator role. Right?"

"Absolutely," Thomas nods. "Scrooge was viewing himself as an independent observer, much like you are looking at Figure 4. When you stand apart and observe the inner conflict of the Triangle of Duplicity, you step into the spectator role. In the same way we are looking at the diagram, we must keep the conflicts that live in the Triangle of Duplicity in consciousness for as long as possible. This is like choosing to stay in the psychological pressure cooker, or to put it mildly, purposely staying in a psychological hothouse like this dive workshop. The process of staying aware of and present to our inner duplicities takes an enormous amount of up-front psychological energy, but our ability to perform this type of psychological work will increase. Staying present to the inner conflict is the most accurate description of psychological work and psychological growth that I know of.

"This brings us to the questions, 'What is the actual *mechanism* of deep personal change?' And, 'How does deep personal change actually happen?' Deep change happens through an inner dialectic process that synthesizes the opposing views into a shared paradigm and allows all the complexes of the personality to survive. It is a shared paradigm that all the complexes of the personality can support and buy into.

"I want to use another thought experiment to illustrate what I mean by a shared paradigm. Remember how I used an outer company as an analogy to describe an inner psychological company of the Inner People? Now I want to use an outer dialectic process that you can use in your interpersonal relationships as an analogy to describe the inner dialectic of deep personal change.

"Please bear with me for a minute, if it sounds like I'm teaching a college level course in psychology," Thomas smiles. "Carl Rogers first developed the notion of empathic understanding as a psychotherapeutic method for removing the barriers to authentic interpersonal communication and as a key to developing deep and fulfilling relationships. For Rogers, our tendency to judge, evaluate, to approve (or disapprove of) what other people say, and of who they are, was the greatest barrier to interpersonal communication and relationships.[16] The antidote for these barriers to communication was to develop empathic understanding of the other person.

"Empathy is defined as seeing a situation, or disagreement, from the other person's point of view—walking a mile in their shoes. Developing empathy means we have to learn to really listen to what people are saying to us and understand their personal meaning and what the situation means to them. When the person that we have been arguing with really feels heard and understood, this empathic understanding releases powerful forces of change deep within that person. My experience in relationships has been that when I really listen to someone, when they really feel heard by me, and respected by me for who they are, what they think, and how they feel, they become more open to understanding my point of view as well. The empathic exchange on both parts produces the power of change within both people."

Lindsey volunteers, "I have experienced what you're talking about when dealing with deep, bitter, long-standing employee-supervisor disputes. When either person begins to listen to the other with empathy and the other person feels *heard,* the level of hostility and conflict decreases visibly and the two people are often able to talk about solutions to their problems, and sometimes even salvage the relationship."

"Exactly," Thomas says. "Just like the examples that Lindsey and Maggie gave us before, the hostile and negative energy begins to disappear and we experience the exhilarating psychological energy that is freed-up for constructive things in the relationship to unfold. The negative energy that was wasted only minutes earlier to defend our mutual positions can be redirected to do the positive tasks of relating to each other and moving on with the relationship.

"When we see two people caught in a battle of enormous psychological energy, we are often witnessing an *externalization* of conflict from each person's Triangle of Duplicity into the arena of the interpersonal relationship. For example, a man who argues with his wife is often in conflict with his own Shadow Self or Inferior Self, as is the woman who argues with her husband. But even if people succeed in developing a shared paradigm between them, empathic understanding about externalized interpersonal conflict does not necessarily synthesize the inner opposing views of the Triangle of Duplicity within each of those people.

"But," Thomas asks, "what happens when we recognize the conflict as an *internal* battle within the Triangle of Duplicity of both parties and apply the process of empathic understanding? My experience has been that we gain a window into the fundamental nature of deep change and the overall healing process of the human personality. Much like a dialogue between people, the Conscious Self must learn to see the ideas and attitudes of the Inner People and the Unconscious Self *from the Unconscious's Perspective*. The Conscious Self must learn to sense how the Inner People feel about an issue and see the world from their perspective. In other words, the Conscious Self must empathically relate with how the Inner People have been repressed, locked out of consciousness, and offended by its arrogant strangle-hold on consciousness. Only when the Inner People feel heard and respected to the point where some of their views are integrated into the Conscious Self's paradigm, will the battle begin to cease. Then positive psychological energy will be *freed-up* through the synthesis of opposites. It is this freed-up psychological energy that can be redirected to productive activities of the personality, and give us the strength to discover who we are in the second half of life.

"Judgment, evaluation, and criticism are the biggest barriers to interpersonal communication." Thomas pauses for effect.

These words are suddenly pounding in Dan's head. That's all he ever did, was judge, evaluate, and criticize. The inner nudging of the Unconscious Self confirms Dan's sense that empathic understanding is a kind of antidote for what has caused problems for Dan all his life. The medicine that will cure the disease of judgment is for Dan to start seeing situations from the other's point of view—to metaphorically walk a mile in their shoes. If Dan really wants a "cure" for his ailing relationships, he needs to learn to really listen to what people are saying to him, then respond in such a way that they feel heard and understood. He needs to use empathic understanding to make sure that people feel respected for who they are, what they think, and how they feel. He realizes he needs to stop resenting people for not following the rules, by moving into the spectator role of empathic inquiry and admitting his own duplicity of not wanting to follow the rules. Dan hammers mercilessly on rule breakers, because he is one. We always hate what we secretly are.

Dan sees that empathic understanding is a way for him to get serenity in his relationships and in his life. When he spots a flaw or problem in other people, or in the world around him, Dan realizes he needs to learn how to not judge, to leave it alone. He needs to stop picking at what's "wrong" like a little boy picking at a scab, or like a dog nipping at an injured leg. Dan is beginning to see that he will need to start taking the world as it is, without reacting to it, or rejecting it based on his own internal black and white standards of right and wrong. He needs to learn to "listen with his eyes and his gut" for what is really happening with other people, not cramming them into his prepackaged mold of evaluation and judgment.

Thomas continues, "How long must we endure the psychological pressure of the inner dialectic before the synthesis happens? The short answer is, 'It takes as long as it takes.' The long answer is, 'It takes as long as it takes.'" Several people chuckle at this as Thomas presses on. "Depending on the issue and the person, it could take days, weeks or years. Sometimes there is never a full and complete synthesis where the battle totally ceases. It can be compared to the process involved in such things as:

- Grieving after the death of someone you love,
- Coming to grips with the pain of being laid off,
- Adjusting to the freedom that comes when we leave a bad marriage,
- Processing the feelings of being betrayed by a close friend, or
- Working through the suicide of a friend who seemed to have everything going for them."

"Yeah," Bethany comments. "I wonder how long it took that farmer husband to work through his feelings about his wife killing herself with his shotgun in her own nicely-scrubbed kitchen?"

The group nods in assent with Bethany's comment. Thomas acknowledges her, then takes a step toward the teaching table, and continues, "When you stay present to these deep emotions in your heart and your gut, they beat against your inner vessel and widen your perspective on life. When you hold them in the space of consciousness, they produce a sweet-sorrowful sense that we really can find some meaning in suffering. Our ability to vessel and contain these types of enormously strong emotions causes us to be motivated by the Basic Trust that we will survive psychologically as a whole person.

"One day we wake up and the battle is over. Sometimes we feel that we have crossed some inner line and the energy just isn't there for us anymore. The inappropriate levels of energy that have bound us are cut in half, or are completely gone. We confront a situation that has troubled us a hundred times before, and the inappropriate level of energy does not appear on cue like it used to. This kind of deep change *happens to us* when we allow the inner dialectic to run its course and wait for the opposing views within us to synthesize.

"You can't get something for nothing," Thomas shrugs his shoulders. "You must learn how to free up the psychological energy that you formerly squandered on Defense Mechanisms, Unintended Consequences, toxic relationships, and spring-loading in order to get deep personal change. This is why traditional approaches to self-help don't work. They normally exhort us to try harder and think positively, which requires us to muster more psychological energy that is already in short supply."

Thomas relaxes his posture and smiles. "When the battle within the Triangle of Duplicity subsides, there is a rush of excess psychological energy that is freed up. Our interest in life is piqued and we no longer have to psychologically rob Peter to pay Paul just to get through the day. We are alive, maybe for the first time in our lives."

Everyone is taken aback when Rick seems to come alive and interrupts with, "Well, what about when you dream about a battle with wild animals? How does *that* kind of conflict get synthesized?"

Thomas is wondering if this is a personal experience Rick has had, or whether he is just trying to derail the discussion. Either way, Rick's question turns out to be a nice opening to an important aspect about the nature of the unconscious. Thomas decides to entertain the question, which is probably much more than Rick anticipated. "Let me make a crucial note of dimensionality. The unconscious sometimes chooses to reveal its side of the story to the dreamer in symbols that take on human form. These instances come the closest to viewing the dialectic as the process of the Unconscious Self mediating, with empathic understanding between the Conscious Self and the Inner People.

"But often, the Unconscious Self uses archetypal symbols that are only partly human, or non-human as Rick suggests, in some dreams. While describing the attributes of the Unconscious Self in the human-like terms of a mediator of the conflict is helpful, we must always remember that the archetypes are raw, primitive, collective, animal, instinctual energy that care nothing for us as individuals. The archetypes do not *care* whether we are consumed or destroyed by the demands of the calling to discover who we really are.

"When the partly human or non-human archetypal symbols reveal their compensatory side of the story, it is still a *dialectic interaction, but it is not a discussion* between disagreeing parties. The archetypes often communicate messages that flow from the depths of the mystery of the biological-psychological interface with the power of an artesian eruption. When a dreamer is thrust into a scene where he is participating in a battle with more than life-sized stone chess pieces—like Harry Potter and his friends—or fleeing from the Dark Riders—like Frodo in Tolkien's *Lord of the Rings*—he is forced against his will to interact with the raw, unmitigated power of these archetypal symbols. But there is no way for the dreamer to *reason* with these elements of the unconscious and there is certainly no way to *talk it out* with archetypal symbols."[17]

"I'll bet that some of the images in the stories you just named originally came from archetypal symbols that appeared to the writers in dreams," says Lindsey.

Thomas raises his eyebrows, "You may be right, Lindsey. Most writers who produce stories like those mentioned live very close to the unconscious."

Thomas points over the railing of the boat to the beach of the island, and says, "Like the waves pounding on the sand, these people live at the metaphorical shoreline between the ground of consciousness and waters of the deep archetypal unconscious.

"As dreamers we must learn to *fear* the unconscious when we are forced to dialectically interact with snarling tigers; charging buffalo; primitive sharks; raging bears; wild stallions; disgusting insects; animated trees that attack us; or various monsters. These archetypal creatures are determined to have their way with us psychologically, and it's not possible for us to stop them. All we can do is develop the psychological consciousness required to ensure that the archetypes do not take over our facilities when we least expect, like the Inner People do. When the model of empathic understanding in personal interactions is calibrated with non-human aspects of the human personality, we come to understand that the *dialectic* process is an interaction, but it is not always a *discussion*. When the dreamer is led down into deep underground caverns or secret tunnels under a fortress or castle where they are the only human thing along the way, they start to understand the true nature of the depths of the human personality.

"Fearing the unconscious is like the healthy fear of the ocean that every diver must have. I'm not talking about the kind of Basic Fear that we had on the downward bubble dive, I'm talking about a fear that is more about *respect*. Every now and then I hear over-confident divers saying, 'How could someone possibly die in a diving accident?' I always tell them to get that thought out of their minds because not having a healthy fear of the dangers of diving *is* the first step toward having a diving fatality."

As he is talking, Thomas walks over to where his dive gear is lashed to the boat with a bungee cord, puts his hand on the top valve of the air tank, turns back to the group, and says, "I have two points for you to reflect on. First, connect to some emotions that you feel deeply and try to view them as belonging to the Inner People, then objectively step outside of them the same way you viewed Figure 4 as a spectator. Second, connect to an experience that you've had where the battle raged over some issue, then one day it was just gone and you felt the release of freed-up psychic energy. Are there any questions? If not, then let's go diving."

∿∿∿∿

Kirsten was standing at the whiteboard posted on the main deck, drawing out the underwater topography of the dive site as the group, including Joel, pulled their neoprene wetsuits over their warm bodies. Minutes later they had rolled off the two tenders and were once again alone in the world that was so unlike the one they lived in above the water.

Nitrogen has an interesting effect on people when they go too deep. The air that divers breathe from their tanks is just like the air above the surface of the water, 21 percent oxygen, 78 percent nitrogen, and 1 percent inert gasses. The oxygen gets metabolized into the blood stream, but nitrogen just dissolves into the fatty tissues around the nerve cells and builds up in the diver's body. Surfacing with too much nitrogen left in your body is how people get decompression sickness, it's how they get "the bends."

But nitrogen has another interesting effect on people. While the effect varies from diver to diver, most people going to depths of one hundred feet or more experience the narcotic effects of nitrogen, colloquially known as "getting narced." When a diver is narced, the effect is similar to being intoxicated—like having a second glass of wine. It's a common scuba joke how narced divers pull their regulators out of their mouths so they can kiss the fish on the lips. On the serious side, getting narced lowers a diver's sense of danger and their respect for safety measures, consequently putting themselves or others into jeopardy at depth.

It's also interesting how the depths of the unconscious have a narcotic effect on people. It happens in two ways. First, when one of the Inner People or an archetype takes control of the facility and drives the Conscious Self down into the depths of the unconscious, we become obsessed, taken over, consumed with intoxifying levels of psychological energy and powerful emotions. Being at depth in the unconscious distorts our judgment and perspective about our relationships and life. And it is while being at psychological depth that we say and do things that we end up regretting for the rest of our lives. This is why most people stay "shallow" in life and don't go into the deep places of their personality.

But consciously learning to *Dive In* to the depths of the unconscious and explore the full scope of your personality teaches "inner divers" how to handle being psychologically narced. Since every person's tolerance is different, inner divers learn at what depth they start to feel intoxicated, they know what their personal depth limit is, and they learn not to perform complicated tasks at depth because that's when you begin to feel the narcotic effect most strongly. Knowing and diving the depths of the unconscious builds our tolerance and enables us to function at psychic and emotional depth. So when an inner diver is taken over by the Inner People or an archetype, and is pulled from the surface of conscious life to the depths where the narcotic effects are most powerful, they become stronger because of their experience of doing psychological work. Experienced inner divers are not so easily drawn in, and become increasingly skilled at sidestepping and not identifying with the intoxicating effects of the emotions of the Inner People.

SESSION 3: RESTORING OUR FREEDOM TO CHOOSE

Mike rings the bell at 3:00 P.M. to start the next session, as Kirsten gives Joel a private dive brief on the dive the two of them are about to make. Thomas sets down his markers on the flip chart, turns to the group, and steps closer to the teaching table. "We lose our freedom to choose in life so early that we don't even know we've lost anything. By identifying with the Conscious Self by age two or three, we become the prisoner of its filtering process and preferences about life. The *central claim* of this session is that developing skill in the first three Competencies *gives us our freedom back*. What we gain is the freedom to choose how we'll respond to any situation, rather than just responding mechanically out of the stock set of responses of the Conscious Self. In the big picture, we gain the freedom to live our lives the way we want for the very first time. This allows us to begin discovering who we really are and to experience that self who never existed, the Emergent Self.

"This loss of freedom that happens by age two or three has very tangible results in that we develop automatic psychological responses. These automatic responses produce habits that fall below the surface of consciousness, and we live out our lives on *automatic pilot*.

"When the battle within the Triangle of Duplicity begins to sub- side and the obfuscating dust that has clouded the inner vision of the personality settles, we see our psychological landscape with new clarity for the very first time. As the Inner People are allowed to have more facility time, *they grow up* and act like mature, productive aspects of the personality, rather than as iconoclasts or rebels who devote all their time and energy to defeating the totalitarian control of the Conscious Self.

"When we answer the calling of the Unconscious Self, follow its guidance, and learn from the inner wisdom of the Four Competencies, this is the fundamental turning point in the inner civil war for control of the personality. There will be many battles to fight after this, but as we move along the path of answering the calling, they become less frequent, and have far fewer consequences on the overall organization, harmony, and unity of the human personality."

Thomas points over the side of the boat and says, "The clear blue water allows us to see the reef structure below the surface. In much the same way, skill in the first three Competencies allows us to see below the surface of consciousness to the causes and motivations of the automatic responses that have kept us prisoners for the first half of life. We know that we are on the road to discovering who we are when we begin to experience three types of freedom from the conflict in the Triangle of Duplicity.

"First, we experience freedom from Unintended Consequences. Formerly, the Conscious Self would choose for us and the Inner People were forced to disrupt these goals and intentions by taking over the facility." Thomas holds up the previously shown Figure 5 as a visual aid. "But as we move further and further upstream, we can catch ourselves in the act of being taken over by the Inner People, rather than looking back on situations after-the-fact. This is a sign of increasing collaboration between the Inner People and the Conscious Self.

"Second, we experience freedom from Defense Mechanisms and being consumed by inappropriate levels of psychological energy. We also become free from distortion and obfuscation of the Defense Mechanisms of the Conscious Self and increasingly recognize when we are caught in the Projection Principle.

"Third, we experience freedom to explore our inner wisdom by encouraging the unconscious to communicate its perspective to us because we respect, listen to, and ultimately value the perspective of the Unconscious Self and the Inner People as an inner hidden treasure. We come to understand the images and symbols in our dreams more clearly so they can reveal powerful guidance about how we discover our destiny, and follow the path of discovering who we are.

"I have added one item for you to reflect on. Ask yourself, 'Which areas do I most desperately need to find inner freedom?' Are there any questions? If not, let's go diving."

Maggie had dropped to about sixty feet and her eyes were riveted to the underwater show of the reef. Maggie had always cared deeply about coming across well and looking good, but she knew that diving was the great equalizer that stripped away the façades of life. On the boat, it was possible to present the image of being an experienced, seasoned, world-traveled diver by having the latest high-end equipment, and talking a good game of where you have been, and the diving you have done. But once you get into the water, the façade is over. The duplicity of big surface talk is often juxtaposed with a diver who lacks the key skills of buoyancy and relaxed breathing. Underwater this can't be hidden—it's there for all to see.

Maggie's concern with "image" forced her to select people for the 360 who she thought would give her the kind of feedback that she wanted, so the majority of the feedback coincided with her view of her Conscious Self. The small amount of negative feedback that she did get, she dismissed as a result of coming from people who really didn't know her. The Enneagram description of Maggie's Triangle of Duplicity seemed to hit close to home on some of the points. But on the one that Thomas claimed went the deepest and could bring the most profound personal growth, the Inferior Self, Maggie looked inside as honestly and introspectively as she could, but she just couldn't connect the descriptions to her personal experience. For example, her Inferior Self was supposed to be the inner person that was frightened, shy, insecure, and passive, preferring to remain invisible and stay out of the spotlight.

Maggie's image of a competitive, bright, image-conscious, achievement-oriented person who always called attention to herself, stood in the spotlight, and excelled at absolutely everything, was supposed to be a cover for this contradictory inner person. The Three Red Flags did more than anything to help her to connect the Triangle of Duplicity to her experience, because she could recall instances where the characteristics of the Inferior Self tried to push their way into the fringe of her consciousness. But somehow these insights were just not enough for her to experience the psychological "click" needed to connect the teaching to her own experience.

But somewhere in this session, where Thomas was discussing how gaining skill in the first three Competencies gave us our freedom back, a sense of the inner awareness of what she had been hearing for the last three days broke into her consciousness. Maggie realized that she never really had the freedom to choose how she would respond to a given situation in life, because she always acted on automatic pilot—a stock set of responses of her competitive, achievement-oriented Conscious Self. Suppose she didn't want to do this? Suppose she wanted to have her own feelings and identity, independent of her achievements and successes? Rather than maintaining the image that she had back at the office, suppose she wanted to reveal J.R. and herself to be the dishonest people that they were?

It's about 6:00 P.M. and Dan and James are hanging out on the upper deck, relaxing with a beer before dinner. They are moving into the fourth day of the trip, and Dan has been a considerate roommate who respects James's boundaries and tries to give him as much psychological space as possible. In addition, from their conversation with Lindsey early this morning James can see that Dan is a person of integrity, struggling with the same kinds of issues that he is.

Following a short pause in the casual conversation they were having about the last dive, Dan takes the discussion to a different level without warning. "Man, I really need to learn this empathic understanding stuff we talked about today. I'm such a hard-ass on my wife and daughter, and I know that many of the people in the business I own just despise me for the same reason. I need to learn to listen to people, and hear what they really say and what they're about without hammering them and judging them before they even get two words out of their mouths."

James is taken aback by the kind of brutal honesty that Dan is showing. His gut tells him to trust Dan, and to respond by disclosing more about himself, too. "I love my wife and children more than life itself," says James. "I need to find my place in this life. I get too bothered sometimes by my past and things I have done. I need to focus more on living from this day forward. I've been on a journey to somewhere and I haven't known where to go or what to do, but it's becoming clearer with this dive workshop."

They share a few more of their concerns, lapse into some more casual conversation about diving, and before they know it, the bell rings for dinner. As Dan and James climb down the steep stairs to the main deck, they both sense that they are common souls who have happened to connect on this trip, and they could probably become lasting friends who stay in contact for a lifetime.

The deep blue tablecloth, dinner candles, wineglasses, and serving plates always transform the teaching table into a place that looks more like a banquet hall than the deck of a ship. Long after everyone has excused themselves from the dinner table, Lindsey and Maggie sit drinking wine and pouring their hearts out to each other. Lindsey feels so naked and exposed by the comments of the 360-degree review, and the Enneagram description of the Triangle of Duplicity, that she is almost ashamed to go back to the office. The workshop has powerfully shown her what some of her issues are, but she is unsure where she should go from here. After a pause to pour their fourth glass of wine, Maggie says, "I realized today how much I live on automatic pilot and how much freedom and autonomy I give up by doing it. I am so sick of playing the game, being on the treadmill with people and life." Then in a way that is honest to the core and contains no arrogance, Maggie says, "It's hard to look the way I do. Every man wants a piece of you. Looking like me gets you places you wouldn't otherwise get, especially with men, and I have played that card long and hard for most of my life. I often win at whatever I'm competing for, but I don't often win honestly." Whether it's the wine, the insight and mood that the workshop creates, or both, Lindsey is deeply moved by Maggie's openness and vulnerability.

Day 4

BACK TO THE FLORES SEA

~~~~~

Competency 4:

Make Three

Commitments

~~~~~

THE DAY BEGINS

The *Explorer* has sailed north and moored off the island of Gili Lawa Darat on the northeast coast of Komodo Island and all on board are preparing for another great day of diving back in the warm waters of the Flores Sea. At breakfast, Joel, Rick, Lindsey, and Bethany are sitting together and comparing notes on what they saw yesterday on the dives. Joel reaches back over the table and picks up the book on marine life to find the name of a particular damsel fish he is trying to explain to Bethany. So long as they steer clear of anything to do with the dive workshop, conversation with Joel flows easily. Once the conversation begins to drift in that direction, Joel makes them feel like trespassers. This has been the tacit discussion format ever since Joel *overtly* dropped out of the workshop and Rick *covertly* dropped out. Keep the conversation on diving with the level of the veneer that typified the first two days, and Joel and Rick fit right in with the group. Stray even a little bit toward talk about the workshop, and Rick tunes out, and Joel generally leaves.

Mike rings the bell to start the first session, and even Thomas has to extract himself from the coffee and discussion in the main cabin.

SESSION 1: A COMMITMENT TO RELATIONSHIPS

Thomas assumes his place next to the flip chart and begins, "As I mentioned earlier in the workshop, the first tendency that most people have to take the inner pressure off when they reach the second half of life is to go after outer change even though the calling really is about deep personal change. However, the Fourth Competency of channeling freed-up psychic energy into Three Commitments is what anchors the inner process of self-discovery to the pedestrian realities of everyday life. While the process of discovering who we are has a sense of transcendence and destiny about it, it is fully rooted and anchored in the realities of the physical world by the Three Commitments. Today, we will cover each commitment in a separate session.

"The First Commitment is to relationships. More specifically, it is a commitment to build a portfolio of relationships that supports us in answering the calling. By the second half of life, we already have a portfolio of relationships and the First Commitment requires us to evaluate them, but what criteria should we use?

"Typically when people evaluate their relationships they use criteria that the Conscious Self used to filter out anxiety, fear, and psychological confusion during the first half of life. More specifically, we see these criteria defined concretely in the interaction of the three Enneagram types within the Triangle of Duplicity. But these criteria are the ones that so often produce portfolios of relationships that inhibit us from answering the calling to discover who we really are. You cannot solve a problem with the same strategies and interpretations that created the problem in the first place."

"In retrospect," says James, "that seems so common sense—why is that concept so hard to understand?"

"Because common sense is not common," Thomas answers, and then presses on. "The *central claim* of this session is that we must use a single, but very different criterion to evaluate the portfolio of relationships that we have in our lives. We must ask, 'To what degree does a given relationship facilitate and support the kind of deep personal change needed to answer the calling to discover who we really are, regardless of how well the relationship maps to the values and beliefs of the Conscious Self?' This criterion will seem counter-intuitive to the Conscious Self because relationships that facilitate and support deep change sometimes create anxiety, fear, and psychological confusion. They don't avoid it, they use these things to create deep change. Relationships that facilitate deep personal change have at least three characteristics.

"First, they often require an enormous *up-front* investment of psychological energy and this up-front investment takes time to pay off, long-term. Relationships that do not require such investments up front may be many things, but normally they are not enablers to change. Relationships that support deep personal change *are work*, but when that work is based on the principles that I have been discussing in this dive workshop, they result in high-leverage, long-term payoff in life.

"Second, they often *require* conflict. Sometimes, they require enormous conflict. Most times it is a mistake to give in to the temptation to leave the relationship just because it produces conflict, without knowing whether the conflict is constructive. Constructive conflict facilitates change and leaving this type of relationship sentences you to take those unresolved issues into your next relationship—one that may be even less supportive of discovering who you are. Destructive conflict undermines the criteria of supporting the deep personal change needed to answer the calling.

"Third, relationships that facilitate change often require us to *purposely* disrupt the equilibrium in a relationship whether they be a friend, sibling, parent, child, or a co-worker. Most people do not choose this path because they are afraid that if they even begin the process, they will open a Pandora's Box and they will never be able to get the lid back on. People who decide to forego dealing with the root causes of conflict in relationships will inevitably build spring-loaded pressure and toxicity in all four quadrants of the Consciousness Matrices of the people involved. The normal response to this is to continue to try to stay on the surface of the relationship, give each other more space, or look on the *bright* side. In some relationships, this situation goes on for a lifetime. In others, it erupts or explodes and almost always ends in tragedy. In the meantime, people wonder why their relationships with their spouses, children, parents, siblings, family, co-workers, or neighbors are problematic.

"But if healthy relationships that facilitate change actually create anxiety, fear, and psychological confusion, how do we tease apart the difference between constructive and destructive conflict? How do we know whether our commitment of enormous amounts of energy will pay off in the end, or lead nowhere but to more and more squandered psychological energy?"

Thomas starts passing around a handout with a diagram of Figure 7 and criteria as he continues to explain.

"When people list all the relationships that they consider to be in their portfolio, the distribution of relationships often follows a 10-10-60-10-10 rule that I use in organizational change initiatives. In any given situation, 20 percent of the people in an organization will be strong supporters of change and 20 percent will be strongly opposed. The sum of the two 10 percent groups on both tails of the distribution is normally set in their beliefs and no amount of persuasion will change their views. My experience is that when we use the single criterion of whether or not relationships facilitate and support change, most people's portfolios of relationships follow a similar distribution, as shown here—" Thomas points to his copy of Figure 7.

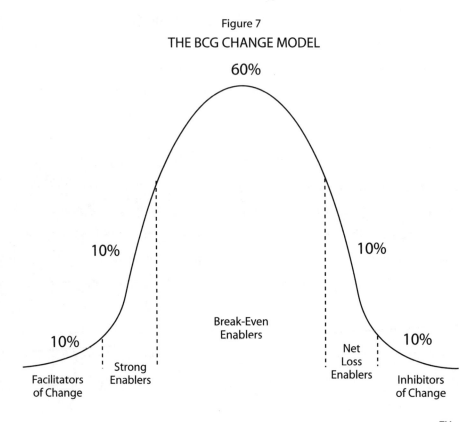

Figure 7
THE BCG CHANGE MODEL

"The connection between organizational change and change in relationships is so similar," says Dan. "But I've never thought about it like that before."

"Well," Thomas replies, "it follows from the assumption that organizations are made of individuals, and consequently they are changed one person at a time. Business processes don't do work, people do. It all comes back to people, relationships, and personality.

"Figure 7 is the BCG Change Model. It shows that 10 percent of the people in our Portfolio of Relationships will be what I call Facilitators of Change and 10 percent will be Strong Enablers of change. On the other tail, 10 percent of the people will be Net-Loss Enablers of change, and 10 percent will be actual Inhibitors of Change.

The remaining 60 percent will be what I call Break Even Enablers of change. The people who fall into the two tail ends of the distribution will be relatively fixed in their views toward us and are not likely to change these views. Let's review the criteria you have in your handout.

"Facilitators of Change are people who:

- See something in us that we do not see in ourselves and mirror it back to us until we do see for ourselves.

- Function in an externalized role of the Unconscious Self or Inner People, in a compensatory manner, regardless of whether they are a spouse, friend, uncle, working associate, neighbor, analyst, or a stranger that you meet on a diving trip to Indonesia. This person carries an archetypal image for us that ignites personal change.

- Model the process of answering the calling in their own lives, and become a concrete example of a person who has become *themselves*. The modeling effect works regardless of whether we actually know the person, or encounter them only in books, movies, or other media."

Thomas is alternately pointing at the flip chart and turning to face the group. "Strong Enablers of change are people who:

- Support us with empathic understanding even when this path would not make sense for them.

- Demonstrate a commitment to us by investing time and psychological energy.

- Demonstrate a commitment to us with financial assistance, or putting their talents and skills at our disposal, or in some other tangible way. Metaphorically and literally, they take us in when we need it most.

- Take a risk for us, use their influence to open doors, or are willing to pay some professional, social, or personal price to support us in our calling.

- Give us psychological energy to answer the calling."

Thomas wipes the sweat from his brow, grabs his water to wet his parched mouth, and continues, "Break Even Enablers are people who:

- Neither give nor take away the attributes of Facilitators of Change or Strong Enablers.

- Keep life on an even keel so we can pursue change.

- Neither give nor take away psychological energy.

- Stay on the surface of the day-to-day business of life so we can pursue change."

Thomas begins to pace the entire length of the teaching table, and becomes more intense in his tone of voice as he says, "Net-Loss Enablers are people who:

- Are *moderately* unconscious of the Unintended Consequences and Defense Mechanisms of the Conscious Self, and who pull us into neurotically fixated interchanges where we rehash the same issues repetitively, without resolution.

- Tend to blur the line between psychological truth and psychological dishonesty: a) by-passing, b) giving inconsistent messages, c) covering up, d) covering up the cover up.[18]

- Consistently take psychological energy, and give little or none in return.

- Say they will support us in answering our calling, but their deeds do not follow their words.

- Chatter mindlessly as a way of venting their anxiety and fears on us.

- Are cynical, negative, glass-half-empty, and who consistently look on the dark side of life and experiences.

- Are legalists who bind us up with the technicalities of "rules" that prevent us from answering the calling.

- Are self-absorbed and narcissistic, and whose consciousness is utterly focused on their wants, desires, interests, pursuits, emotional states, plans, activities, etc.

- Fall victim to one crisis after another. Many of these may even have legitimate reasons attached to them, but regardless of the *reasons* the sheer number of problems and woes are simply overwhelming."

Thomas walks to a point on the deck next to the boat railing. His physical presence becomes less intense, but the tone of his voice is much more serious. "Inhibitors of Change are people who:

- Are almost *totally* unconscious of, and bound by, the Unintended Consequences and Defense Mechanisms of the Conscious Self, and who pull us into neurotically fixated interchanges where we rehash the same issue repetitively, without any hope of resolution.

- Actively and/or passively oppose us in answering our calling. Active opposition is overt and aggressive, while passive aggression is more difficult to detect, but it is still aggression.

- Totally obfuscate and distort the line between psychological truth and psychological dishonesty to the point where the line between sanity and insanity is blurred: a) by-passing, b) giving inconsistent messages, c) covering up, d) covering up the cover up.

- Are emotional vampires who totally drain away our psychological energy, bleed us of the power to live life, and utterly refuse to acknowledge what they do.

- Refuse to take personal responsibility for their actions, emotional life, or any of the characteristics mentioned above. They develop enormously rigid and fundamentalist views that project the causes and blame for issues in life onto the world around them.

◆ Try to give us the impression that we are free, while they try to utterly control our behavior, emotional life, and the other characteristics mentioned above. We only know the extent of the control when we try to gain our freedom."

Thomas walks back to his flip chart and lets a few seconds of silence pass before continuing. "Managing the Portfolio of Relationships means that you should try to migrate people to the left side of the distribution if possible. But you may have to distance yourself from some relationships, and in some cases even terminate them, because of the undermining effects that they have on your attempts to answer the calling. More importantly, after doing this analysis, most people find that they need to bring new people into their lives in order to balance out the distribution and really become the architect, builder, and owner of a Portfolio of Relationships that is of their own choosing. In a sense, you construct your own reality that will mirror back to you the support you need to pursue the process of self discovery. Following the guidance of the Unconscious Self through the Three Red Flags holds out the *hope* that even the damaging effects of Net-Loss Enablers and Inhibitors of Change can be transformed into positive impetus for change by finding *meaning* in the suffering and trauma these people cause in our lives."

Nikki stares off into space as the reality sinks in of how much Todd had tried to be a Facilitator of Change in her life, especially while she was at Yale. She hurts with the deep pain of someone who had gambled that her relationship with Todd would be the lasting one, and had brutally lost because of her own compulsions and blind spots.

Thomas is still talking, "How do we handle people who are consistently Net-Loss Enablers or Inhibitors of Change in our life? Remember what we discussed the first day? There is always another side to the story in a relationship, and others may not even be aware of beliefs held by their Inner People. Whether it's with our parents, children, closest friends, working associates, or neighbors you've known for years, the other side of the story provides valuable information that is ignored at your own peril. Impressions about others that appear on the fringe of consciousness are often how we experience the activity of the Inner People in others. Because people are often unaware of these aspects of their personalities, it is crucial to believe what people *do*, not what they *say*.

"So in some ways, trying to make a decision about a relationship is not unlike what juries do when they piece together the facts of a case using objective evidence, the testimony of people, and their intuitions about what actually happened. As such, when we are attempting to reconstruct what's really going on in a relationship, we do not have to find the absolute truth in the reconstruction. We must simply use the evidence of the Three Red Flags and our intuition to reconstruct the situation *beyond a reasonable doubt*. Trying to establish the *truth* of any situation is a side track at best, and a Defense Mechanism of the Conscious Self.

"My experience with thousands of people in workshops is that naiveté and a lack of psychological development of our instincts and intuitions is a problem that plagues men and woman of all ages. The problem is that people have not sufficiently developed their psychological alarm systems and this allows the Conscious Self to overrule the deeper intuitions that come from the Unconscious Self and the Inner People.

Thomas finds a 3x5 card in his pile of lecture notes. "I want to read a quote to you from Clarisa Pinkola Estes's book, *Women Who Run With the Wolves*. 'In hindsight, almost all of us have, at least once, experienced a compelling idea or semi-dazzling person crawling in through our psychic windows at night and catching us off-guard. Even though they're wearing a ski mask, have a knife between their teeth, and a sack of money slung over their shoulder, we believe them when they tell us they're in the banking business.'"[19]

Some of the people have a good laugh at this, while others look like it struck a little too close to home, as Thomas moves on. "Estes claims that a crucial element in training our intuitions and instincts is asking the right questions. Questions are like the *keys* that open the doors of the psyche, behind which our secrets are hidden and the carnage of self-destruction lies undiscovered. This is why we proceed with an empathic attitude of inquiry and refuse to indulge in the futile judgments and evaluations of the Conscious Self. Estes says we should ask questions like, 'What stands behind? What is not as it appears? What do I know deep in my *ovaries* that I wish I did not know? What of me has been killed or lies dying?' "[20] Thomas motions to the group with his hand. "We ask these questions when someone we're out on a date with says they want to see us again, but does not call, when a friend says she cares but is never there for us, when a parent claims to love us, but does not act in our best interest. We ask these questions when we are uncertain about whether moving to another town, or taking another job, or finding another wife, or going back to school, or investing our life savings in a risky venture, is really what the inner restlessness within us is about."

James asks, "What do you do if these people are in your family?" Others nod their heads in agreement that the most difficult case is when family members are Net-Loss-Enablers, or Inhibitors of Change. "You can't just leave your family."

"Why not?" Thomas retorts. "If family members are abusive, and lack respect for you and your boundaries, or undermine your attempts to answer the calling, why can't you terminate your contact with that person just like you would with any other destructive relationship? It's like divorcing them."

Thomas crosses to his flip chart and turns to Figure 8. "Once we have done the kind of deep introspective analysis we're talking about here, I suggest you use a very concrete tool that I learned from a friend who has been a Facilitator and Strong Enabler of change in my life, Frank Hawkins. The Hawkins Model of Decision-Making asks six simple questions as a way of moving forward in problematic relationships. If you will turn your attention to Figure 8.

Figure 8
**THE HAWKINS MODEL OF
DECISION-MAKING**

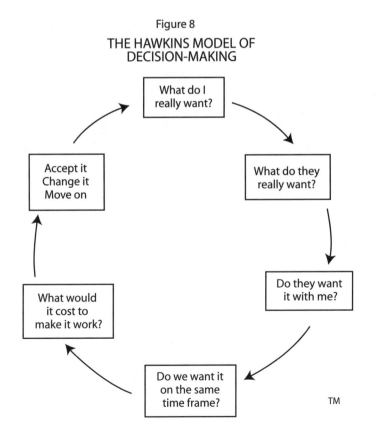

"These six questions can be used to evaluate a relationship, regardless of whether it is someone you are dating, married to, a friend, a family member, a working associate, or a manager in the company you work in. You simply ask:

- What do I really want in the relationship?
- What does the other person want in the relationship?
- Do they want it with me?
- Do we want it on the same time frame?
- What would it cost to make the relationship work—time, energy, money, et cetera?
- Should I accept it, change it, or move on?"

"Sometimes fathers want very different types of relationships with their sons than their sons want. Sometimes managers want very different relationships with their workers than their workers want. Sometimes people both want the same thing, but they do not want it with each other. For example, 'I would really like to get married and have children, I just do not want to do it with you.' It can also be the case that people want the same things and they even want it with each other, but they want it on very different timeframes. For example, 'I may want to hire you into this position, but I cannot do it till next fiscal year, and you need a job now.' Sometimes people want the same things in a relationship, on the same time frame, but they are unwilling to pay the price it would take to have the relationship. Long-distance relationships between lovers, family, friends, et cetera, where people feel pressure to move or change professions, sometimes fall into this category. Based on these questions, the Hawkins Model states that we always have three choices in life:

1. We can accept the way things are,
2. We can try to change them, or
3. We can just move on.

"Deciding to accept or change a situation means that we cycle back to the first question and ask it again. Moving on and away from a relationship may be a temporary situation where we put the relationship on the proverbial *back burner* for some period of time, and then at some time in the future we try to reengage in the relationship by returning to question one. Occasionally, it means that we have to terminate a relationship and remove ourselves from all contact permanently."

"I'm torn by what you're saying," Lindsey says. "It sounds like the idea of *tough love*, which I support, where parents have to tell their children, 'I love you, but you can't do drugs and live here with us.'"

Thomas replies, "The Hawkins Model does not make the decision for you, it says that in the end you only have three choices in life. To use your example, Lindsey, those parents always have these choices—they can accept the fact that their kid is doing drugs, they can try to change him, or they can tell the kid to move on. Quite frankly, I don't know what other realistic alternatives there are in life."

Lindsey and the rest of the group are silent, having no viable response to the view Thomas is presenting.

Looking down toward the deck of the ship, Thomas says, "In some problematic relationships, we struggle, and struggle, and struggle, and struggle some more to make things work. Then one day we wake up in the morning, or we are standing in the shower, or we receive one more put-down in a meeting, and we suddenly realize that we have *crossed some inner line*. The fixated psychological energy is just gone, or we just don't feel like going one more round in the struggle, and the relationship is different. It is almost as if the unconscious has been working on the problem, and simply presents a resolution. Sometimes the relationship is just over. As I mentioned, these relationships are candidates for the back burner, for using time and distance to allow the spring-loading and toxicity in the Consciousness Matrix of both people to re-orient. We can explain our intentions to the other person. We can say that we are willing to entertain the possibility of someday reconnecting through the relationship, but then we move on and go it alone. My experience has been that this type of ruptured relationship can be restored, given enough time and distance, but normally people must draw new lines and boundaries for the new relationship. More times than not, the lines and boundaries that are redrawn are more conservative and probably more appropriate than the original ones. These relationships can actually become deeper than they were originally, but often this takes an enormous investment of psychological energy and time.

"Relationships are objective things that have tangible physical aspects that are part of the interrelated web that we live in. In other words, relationships have houses, cars, bank accounts, pets, children, and other physical things that go along with them. The reality of relationships as *objective things* finds its most powerful support in the fact that these elements of our socially constructed world have to be dismantled and deconstructed when these relationships end. We go different places, we do different things, we move to new houses. We are forced to change our holiday routines, sell or buy cars, take names out of our phone books, stop sending cards and presents at Christmas time, find different jobs, and myriad other changes. These changes are real and objective in the sense that they make a physical difference in our lives and in the lives of the other people involved."

Nikki, who was still hurting about the way Todd had left her, asked, "How do you know when it's time to leave someone? I mean, you can always forgive, or try to smooth things over one more time. When is enough, enough?"

Thomas senses that Nikki has some pain around this issue. "As a general rule, I try never to give up on people entirely, but occasionally we have no alternative. Sometimes people must divorce their spouse, parents, children, manager, or a duplicitous friend because they have crossed some inner line, or because this person has become an enormous Inhibitor of Change. This is probably the most difficult part of making and keeping the First Commitment—the willingness to systematically deconstruct and dissolve relationships that frustrate or work against us in our pursuit of answering the calling to become ourselves. Sometimes, we just have to go it alone because we are bound by the existential reality of freedom and choice. In other words, not making a choice in a toxic, spring-loaded, and dysfunctional relationship is itself a choice. There is no escape from the consequences of our choices, even the choice of not choosing. That's why it always comes down to three choices: accept it, change it, or move on.

"The First Commitment also calls us to become a Facilitator of Change in the lives of other people." Thomas goes on to explain, "The best way that I can think of to describe what I mean by a Facilitator of Change is to recount a story that a friend once told me where someone stepped into this role in her life. Let's call her Amy. Amy grew up in a family where her parents were neurotically fixated in the belief that everything she did, *was a total reflection on them.* Consequently, finding her own sense of self was made difficult or impossible whenever this differed from what they wanted for her. This was especially true when it came to how well she did in school. A good part of the verbal and physical abuse that Amy received while growing up had, 'How well I did in school' as the primary focus. While she was told repetitively by her father, 'You're not stupid, so why don't you do better in school?' his abusive tone always *made her feel stupid* and her poor performance in school became the empirical evidence that placed the label of *stupid* on her own sense of identity. During her high school years, her father took an overdose of sleeping pills following Amy's bringing home a report card with very poor grades. When the father awoke in the hospital and the doctor asked him why he had tried to commit suicide, he told the doctor, 'Because my daughter is failing in school.' She graduated from high school in spite of the nagging fear that she was *stupid*, although this type of emotional baggage can become a self-fulfilling prophecy.

Amy spent the first four or five years after high school making her living as a cocktail waitress, then decided to go to college. She felt functionally illiterate because of the years she had been an under-achiever in school, plus she had been away from reading and study for some years after high school. But she was motivated, some would say driven, to succeed. One day, one of the brightest professors at the college called her into his office, and after swearing her to confidence about the topic for as long as she was in school, he told her the following. 'Amy, you show great promise as a scholar and a teacher. Because of this, I would like to pay your tuition for the remaining time you are here, and give you a monthly book allowance to build a scholarly library.' That person was a Facilitator of Change in Amy's life. He saw something in her that she did not see in herself and he held the mirror up long enough for her to begin to see it on her own. That is what being a Facilitator of Change is all about: looking deeply into people's lives and seeing who they really are. Facilitators of Change look below the surface and the rough edges to the calling that lies beneath. Facilitators of Change search beyond the empirical evidence of how the *system* or the *family* has labeled a person, and hold up a mirror long enough for that person to begin to see their calling for themselves."

"Part of me is shocked and revolted by that story," says Bethany, "yet I see this kind of thing all the time in my line of work—dysfunctional parents trying to live their lives through their kids. Thank God for people like that professor."

The group nods empathically in agreement as Thomas moves on. "We must allow the Unconscious Self to lead us to people, or point out existing relationships where we can become Facilitators of Change or Strong Enablers of change. We must look deeply into people and see in them what they do not see in themselves, then hold the mirror up until they begin to see who they can become. I can hardly imagine a more powerful and meaningful contribution that we can make to the lives of other people."

Thomas's posture indicates he's wrapping up. "There are two things I'd like you to reflect on. First, reflect on the relationships in your life using the single criterion: 'Do they facilitate and support me discovering who I am?' Second, 'How would the people in the 360-degree review evaluate me by this same criterion? Am I a facilitator of deep personal change in their lives?' Okay, are there any questions?"

Dan has already done a quick evaluation in his mind and realizes that he needs to do serious work on his relationship portfolio. Much of the negative energy he feels is of his own making. In his relationship with his daughter, Carol, he is more of an Inhibitor of Change because he resents her not wanting to be involved in the business and relocating to take a job at the Prodigal software company. In mid-thought he hears Thomas's signature line, "Okay, let's gear up and go diving."

For James, many of his problems in life had been about how to relate to, and interact with, people. His underwater reflection revealed to him that his defense had been to just tell everyone to stay away. But now, the deep inner change that he sensed in himself, along with the single criterion for relationships of facilitating and enabling deep personal change, gave him a practical path to move on. More than anything, the distinctions that Thomas discussed early on in the workshop helped to show how black-and-white his thinking was about relationships. Formerly, he had to force people into one of two categories: they either would or would not betray him. And when he had any doubt at all, he just assumed that they would if they could. The distinction of reliability forced him to abandon any notion about the "truth" of whether people would or would not betray him, and instead base his evaluation of people's trustworthiness and the *probability* of them betraying him based on the principle of reliability. Of course, there was always the possibility that people might screw James behind his back, but year after year of consistent, reliably trustworthy behavior made this less and less likely. That was a solution that James could live with.

James's family relationships brought the sense of intimacy and closeness that he so desperately needed. Many nights, he would stare at his sleeping son Jon, now only seven months old, and experience some unspoken part of himself saying, "Heal me, son, heal me." James never fully knew what this experience meant, but he treasured it to the depths of his soul. He realized now how he had always hungered and thirsted for true innocence, the innocence he lost somewhere along the way in life. With the dive workshop, he now knew that more fully experiencing his own wounded sense of innocence was the next step in the life-long journey of self-discovery.

The dive workshop material had also begun to help explain the strange stirrings that went to the depths of James's soul. The teaching somehow touched his inner sense of restlessness with a promise that he would find a way to live a life of meaning and contribution. James had already begun an inner journey without knowing where he was going, and he now had new insight, direction, and a sense of purpose, that he could move beyond the Triangle of Duplicity that had so dominated his life. James longed to continue his path of self-discovery and find that self he had never been before. Being a diver was like being an amphibian who could move in the space between two worlds. James was experiencing that space in-between with great power and intensity.

SESSION 2: A COMMITMENT TO MAKING A DIFFERENCE IN LIFE

The dive ends about 10:40 A.M. and the crew brings the two tenders up onto the main boat, hoists the anchor, and the *Explorer* begins the short sail north to the island of Gili Lawah Laut. By heading in this direction, the ship has already begun the long journey back to Bali. With the boat moving effortlessly through the flat calm waters of the Flores Sea, at 11:00 A.M. Thomas rings the bell to start the next session for the day.

Once everyone, except Joel, is seated, Thomas begins, "The Second Commitment is to making a difference in life. This is not about joining the Peace Corps or becoming a worker at an inner-city Salvation Army rescue mission. It is about making a commitment to your own creativity. When creativity is cashed out in observable ways, the results are real and make a physical difference in the world. The *central claim* of this session is that the process of discovering who you are is a process of integrating unconscious and opposing elements with consciousness, and organizing, harmonizing, and unifying the fragmented complexes of the personality into a whole. The Unconscious Self facilitates this psychic transformation in ways that have many parallels with the creative process.

"To begin with, a focus on, and knowledge of, a body of knowledge is a prerequisite for generating creative ideas. It is unlikely that a person will find a creative solution to a robust problem in mathematics or physics if they have little or no knowledge in these bodies of knowledge. Creativity in music, art, dancing, sports, or other areas, presupposes competency in these areas. Without competency, a person will most likely develop uninformed, mediocre imitations of what other people have done. It should come as no surprise that people are normally creative in areas in which they have been highly trained and worked diligently and consciously for extended periods of time.

"Creativity and making a difference in life are inextricably bound in the sense of the distinction we used earlier that something is real only when it makes a physical difference. Having creative ideas is necessary, but not sufficient to make a person *truly* creative. The truly creative person moves beyond ideas and concretizes their insights into something that can be *publicly observable* by one of the five senses. If creative insights are not instantiated in a way that is publicly observable, then nothing new has been *created* and there has been no real creativity. To be truly creative means, by definition, to give birth to something that previously *did not exist*. In the parlance I have been using, if creativity makes a physical difference, then it's real. If it makes no physical difference, then it's not real. True creativity can only be seen in the *creative act*, and these creative acts must, at least in principle, be capable of being known by others. The greatest difference between a person who *seems* to have creative talent and the *truly* creative person, is their ability to incarnate creative insights into the arena of publicly observable representations, be they equations, technological innovations, or a painting that captures the imagination of an entire generation."

James inserts, "I've always said that there were two kinds of people in life: *pretenders*, and *contenders*. Sounds like people who have creative ideas, but can't cash them out into something real are pretenders—creative day-dreamers."

"Yes," Thomas chuckles, "the truly creative person *links* invisible archetypal symbols to publicly observable representations in such a way that the invisible nature of the archetypal symbol is made visible in the representation. In physics, this might involve identifying deeper underlying symmetries between seemingly unrelated phenomena like Newton's unification of terrestrial and celestial mechanics, or high-energy physics development of the Standard Model of the universe. In music, it might be Jimi Hendrix's ability to aurally represent the traumatic collective ethos of the Vietnam War in his Woodstock rendition of the *Star Spangled Banner*. In movie productions, like *A Beautiful Mind*, we witness invisible archetypal symbols that represent the twenty-first century's collective resonance of people who don't know what reality is, or whether or not they are still sane.

"Not only is the world changed in the creative process because something new has come into existence, but the person who is the channel, or conduit of the creative act is also changed in the process. The channeling of deep archetypal symbols *through* a person and *into* a concrete representation is an incredibly powerful process of transformation. In the creative process, the Conscious Self allows itself to be pushed aside and the psychological energy of an archetypal symbol takes possession of a portion of consciousness and the person's body. The worldview of the unconscious is then channeled into existence in the world by using the creative person's physical body and competencies. When the creative person has the psychological strength to tolerate this inner tension, it often results in a truly creative expression. When they cannot, they cross the line into neurosis or psychosis. This is why creativity and genius have long been associated with insanity."

"That was precisely why the movie, *A Beautiful Mind*, was so confusing in the first part," Maggie said. "I found myself wondering, 'Is John Nash so brilliant that he sees things us mere mortals don't, or is he just crazy?'"

"As it turns out, he was both," Thomas frowns empathically. "To reflect back on our earlier discussion about the Inner People and multiple personalities, when John Nash believed that the projections of his Inner People were out in the world, he was viewed as psychotic, put in a mental hospital, and given electric shock treatment. Once he understood that these Inner People were really inside of him, and that they only had power over him when he acted out what they wanted him to do, which is tantamount to them gaining control of his facility, he was on the road to psychological health.

"So let's return to our topic, 'A life lived making a physical difference in life is a life where we help to *create reality* and leave a legacy.' A tangible evidence of this kind of creativity is being a Facilitator of Change in the lives of others. This multiplies the difference in life that spreads out like an enormous network of change agents. The legacy that you leave behind is a path filled with changed lives."

Lindsey has become increasingly aware that most people can't be fooled by her façade of servant-hood. The illusion of being able to conceal her duplicity and flattery by keeping it out of consciousness is ineffective because the takeovers by the Inner People have a very real negative effect in her life and relationships. Thomas's words about deep change are pounding in her head with an urgency and power that is almost disorienting. Lindsey finds the prospect of allowing the Unconscious Self to integrate her dark side with consciousness to be terrifying and a challenge to the person she has always consciously been. But the hope of having her increasing sense of psychic fragmentation harmonized into a psychic whole is a powerful motivator for overcoming her fear. It holds the hope of building her sense of self on a humility that comes from a complete understanding of all parts of her personality, rather than the façade of being such a special, giving servant to all, a role she has begun to reject about herself. The single criterion for relationships of people being facilitators and enablers of deep personal change challenges her deeply entrenched pattern of giving to people in order to get something in return. But what Lindsey finds most enticing is the prospect of beginning to walk the path of discovering who she really is by focusing on her own creative abilities, rather than finding so much of her own identity in the relationships and people in her life.

Lindsey raises her hand, "Thomas, can you tell us more about the way the creative process actually works in everyday experience?"

Thomas nods, "Good question, Lindsey, I was just getting to that. In terms of describing the creative process, Figure 9 is an adaptation of a model developed by Graham Wallas that mirrors many peoples' experience of the creative process."[21] Thomas reaches over and flips to the next page.

Figure 9

THE CREATIVE PROCESS

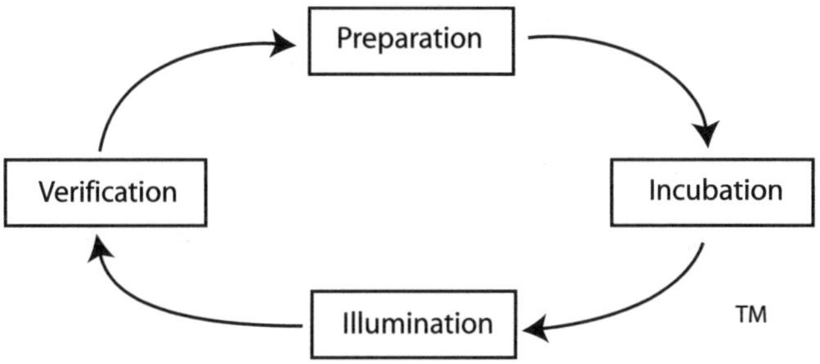

"We already discussed the step of Preparation where people must develop a certain level of expertise in a domain in order to make contributions there. Many people have had the experience of beliefs, the solutions to robust problems, and creative ideas just emerge into consciousness *intact* as the result of unconscious processes. The emergence of such beliefs or solutions is not under the direct control of the Conscious Self, but it does not just happen by accident. As Wallas's model suggests, it often occurs after a person spends an extended period of time thinking about a particular problem and then comes to an immovable roadblock about a path forward. When a person hits this type of roadblock, if they simply occupy themselves with other unrelated activities, or just get a good night's sleep, this begins the process of Incubation. After some unspecified period of time, the answer to the problem often emerges into consciousness as if unconscious processes continued to work on it long after *we* stopped consciously thinking about it. This is the step of Illumination."

"It's like a *Eureka* experience, when a light goes on in your head," says James.

"Correct!" Thomas gives a thumbs-up. "From our discussion on the third Red Flag—the Unconscious's Perspective—we know that this is exactly what happens. Sometimes, the Inner People use their own data, strategies, and perspective and propose a solution that was a stroke of genius to us way up in the space of consciousness. Other times, the Conscious Self finds itself in the uncomfortable position of having a solution or a belief emerge into consciousness that it has previously rejected, or that it is diametrically opposed to as even possible. Finally, when the creative idea has been cashed out into some publicly observable way for others to see, the final step of Validation occurs where people recognize, and are able to use, our creative work in their lives. We help to create reality by making a physical difference in life."

"Sounds good, eh?" Thomas grins. "When do we begin?" The divers smile back.

"Ironically," Thomas continues, "people are often afraid of their own creative abilities. My experience has taught me that people do not make and keep the Second Commitment because they are *terrified* by the power, and unpredictability, of their own creative process. I often hear leaders in organizations lament the lack of creativity of their workers. I have likewise heard this complaint from college professors, priests, government officials, and even parents of children. If so many people lament the fact that they, or others they interact with, are not more creative, and if creativity is such a valued and sought-after commodity in life, and it's a tool of personal transformation, why doesn't society produce more truly creative individuals? There are two main reasons that are equally self-defeating. First, people fear *their own* creative impulses.

They are afraid of what would happen if they really just *let go*. People are afraid to discuss a creative idea if it goes against their spouse's, parent's, or boss's view of the world. People are afraid to be shamed by producing what *they* view as creative work, only to have *others* mock or dismiss it. Whether at home, in the office, in church, or in a discussion with a neighbor, people are afraid to be criticized, laughed at, dismissed as incompetent because of their creative ideas or their creative work. This might in turn result in adverse affects in their personal relationships or their professional life."

Thomas steps under the bright blue tarp to get out of the sun. "More times than not, the truly creative individual will have to go *against* another person's paradigm, the party line at the office, at home, or myriad other contexts that *stifle and kill creativity*. Consequently, exercising creativity demands tremendous courage. Many times it is easier to simply conform than to buck other people's views of reality or the *system*. When we *knuckle under* to people's attempts to kill our creativity, the Inner People, from whom the creative act so often comes, suffer a brutal inner blow that stays with us. No wonder the unconscious views the Conscious Self as the one who sells out, the one without courage, or the one who has no integrity. It's no wonder that the Inner People rise up against the Conscious Self with *rage*, a rage that the Conscious Self cannot comprehend.

"The second reason why society does not produce more creative people is the fear *of the creative person herself* by the established social structures. Society harbors a timeless fear of creative people like artists and scientists. These are the people who challenge and threaten to deconstruct the status quo. Society fears such people because they breed a kind of insurgence that social orders have a difficult time managing or destroying."[22]

Thomas folds his arms in front of him, and takes a deep breath.

233

"It is no accident that the saint and rebel are often the same person, separated only by time. Joan of Arc was a rebel when they burned her at the stake. Martin Luther King was a rebel when he stood up for the rights of black people. Socrates was a rebel who led the youths of Athens astray with his teachings. Today, these people are revered as major contributors to Western civilization or even as saints. The rebellion of the creative person leads to a spirit of *insurgence*. More times than not, the insurgence of the creative person is much more than a mere *intellectual* battle about one view or another. Creative insurgence is frequently accompanied by a tremendous intensity of affect and even *rage* against the *system* as it currently is. Unbeknownst to the people who lament the lack of creative people, this *is exactly* what creative people do. Society fears creative people and creative people know that society fears them. Creative people often know that they are on a collision course with repressive and often violent and coercive forces of society, but their inner rage makes it difficult or impossible to simply accept things *as they are*."

Thomas pulls one of the empty chairs from around the teaching table, sits to rest his tired feet, and presses on, "There are three questions that I'd like you to reflect on. First, 'Do I recognize the elements of the creative process in my own life?' Second, 'What are the current channels and outlets that I use to channel my creativity?' Third, 'What other channels might I explore, either new ones or channels I used long ago, even back in childhood?' Are there any questions?"

Bethany raises her hand and says, "I see some connection between the Four Competencies and the creative process you mapped out, but I can't quite put it into words."

"Good observation," Thomas says. "This is what I meant when I said that the Unconscious Self facilitates the psychic transformation through our own creative processes. In the same way the process of creativity integrates unconscious insights into consciousness, the bottom line of using the Four Competencies is to integrate the unconscious with consciousness, and with the goal of psychological wholeness of the personality. Okay, are there other questions or comments?" Thomas sees lights going on in people's heads—the presence of creativity, of minds opening, and new connections snapping into place is powerfully bonding the group into a synergistic whole. "Okay, let's go diving."

As the two groups of divers rolled backwards off the tenders into the water, the overall perspective of the reef was a magnificent image of color, elegance, and teeming life. Dan settled in at a depth of about fifty feet and moved closer to the reef. He realized that there was a complexity to reef life that was staggering. He was hovering above an enormous piece of stag horn coral, and the fish swam in and out, and clustered around it because it was their home. They chased each other, then floated with the current, then chased each other again. It was almost like this one piece of coral was the marine equivalent to the neighborhood where Dan lived.

The notion of *linking* the deep archetypal patterns of her personality to her actions and making a difference in life crystallized the notion in Maggie's mind of living a life that was inner-directed, not based on external criteria and standards of success and achievement. Rather, she could be inwardly guided and learn the internal wisdom of the Unconscious Self, regardless of what the standards and values of the social mirror were. In the case of quitting her job, when she listened carefully she already knew what the guidance of the Unconscious Self was. Thomas's distinction early in the workshop about reliability enabled her to begin to make more sense of the life she had lived in the Conscious Self. The fact that there was no black and white "truth" in life was precisely how she lived a life of deceit and lying without ever having to admit it—it was just a different spin, it wasn't really a "lie" per se. Her entire inner and outer life had been built on this axiom. Given the fact that the best we could hope for was an inter-subjective agreement of people agreeing to hold a shared paradigm, Maggie could strive to never misrepresent things again by creating an impression in others that she knew to be misguided. The prospect of linking the wholeness of her personality to the way she actually lived gave her a sense of authenticity and reality that she had never had. From this day forward, she would commit herself to making a difference in the world by making a commitment to her own creative abilities.

SESSION 3: A COMMITMENT TO EFFECTIVE AGING

It's three o'clock and the Indonesian sun is pounding down on the blue tarp that covers the main deck of *Explorer* as Mike rings the bell. By this time in the dive workshop, the ringing of the bell to start the next session has become almost a Pavlovian ritual that calls people from every part of the ship. Thomas is standing at his flip chart listening to a point that Bethany is making to Lindsey about something that she'd realized in the last session. Thomas is pleased that people are getting as much out of it as they are. That's what gives him a sense of meaning and making a contribution in life.

He begins with, "The Third Commitment, to Effective Aging, really anchors the process of discovering who we are to the realities of everyday life. Most people experience the calling to discover who they are in the second half of their life. This period is also when many people become more concerned about the issues associated with Effective Aging. They begin to learn that it's one thing to live long. It's quite another to live well. Living long and living well as biological and psychological beings is a key element in answering our calling.

"The common perception is that longevity of life is almost exclusively about the difference between sickness and health. The inference is that if our lives are free from disease, then we are living well. In addition, recent advances in the discipline of genetics and in the medical field have led to a myopic focus on the genetically transmitted aspects of contracting diseases and having medical problems. There is an increasing body of knowledge that shows that the genetic predisposition powerfully influences the health problems that people have. But this body of knowledge focuses strictly on the biological side of the biological-psychological interface. Two key elements to disease avoidance are proper diet and a regular exercise program, particularly aerobic exercise. While proper diet and exercise are *necessary,* they're not *sufficient* to produce Effective Aging. The world is full of people who are disease-free, yet suffer from the kind of lack of meaning and purpose in life that discovering who they are brings. Effective Aging focuses primarily on the psychological and social aspects of the biological-psychological interface, where the hamburger you ate for lunch becomes the psychological energy to live life."

Thomas walks over to the teaching table, grabs a glass of water, and wets his parched mouth. "One body of research that undermines the common perception that longevity of life is about the difference between sickness and health, and shows how we can mitigate genetic factors, is the work of Hans Selye on stress. Selye's research suggests that people respond to stress in three stages that he calls the General Adaptation Syndrome (G.A.S.), also known as the biological stress syndrome. The three stages are: a) the alarm reaction, b) the stage of resistance, and c) the stage of exhaustion. Studies on the combination of the three phases showed that the body's ability to adapt to stress— adaptation energy—is finite. In other words, the body's ability to react to and resist stress along the biological-psychological interface can last only so long before it is exhausted."[23]

Thomas stretches, trying to relax almost on cue with the material he's teaching. "Much like any machine that gradually wears out even if it has adequate fuel, the human organism suffers from continuous wear-and-tear due to stress. The three stages of the G.A.S. are analogous to the three stages of aging: childhood, adulthood, and senility. Selye claims that there is a close relationship between work, stress, and aging. Stress is a *cumulative* thing that adds up to the sum of all the individual stressful incidents that we experience over a lifetime. Increases in stress actually *accelerate* the aging process on a biological level—we wear our bodies out with stress.

"For Selye, stress is not just nervous tension and it is not something to be avoided, because some of it comes from pleasurable, positive experiences where we have succeeded at something we desired over a long period of time. Rather, Sclye's studies showed that it was immaterial whether a stressor was pleasant or unpleasant. What mattered was the intensity of the demand made upon the adaptive capacity of the body. From his view, stress becomes a new concept of mental and physical illness that is defined as the rate of wear and tear on the body caused by life. The studies showed that not only can we overcome the harmful effects of stress, but we can learn to use stress to our own advantage."

"That's why I like diving," Dan asserts. "It's about the only thing in life that really relaxes me."

Thomas smiles in agreement and moves on, "Another study that undermines common perceptions about aging is a Macarthur Foundation Study that shows that even genetically preprogrammed risk factors such as high blood pressure, blood fat levels—cholesterol—and triglycerides, lung function, mental sharpness, and pseudodiabetes of aging can be modified by what they call *successful aging*. The three components of successful aging are: a) avoiding disease, b) engagement with life, and c) maintaining high cognitive and physical functions."[24]

Thomas moves to the ship's railing and leans back to take some of the load off his feet. "In fact, one of the most radical findings that the study produced was the fact that the older one becomes, the less important genetic predisposition becomes and the more important the three factors of successful aging become. In other words, the older we become, the less genetic factors seem to count when all three components of successful aging are combined. The findings that genetic factors can be mitigated are also supported by the results of a study that claims that you can reduce your risk factors for diseases that come from genetic influences by changing your lifestyle to match your blood type."[25]

Thomas walks back to the flip chart, turns the page and points to a list of five items. "The study gives personalized blood-type prescriptions and recommendations for such things as:

a.   lifestyle management,

b.   coping with stress and maintaining emotional balance,

c.   maximizing health,

d.   overcoming disease, and

e.   fighting the effects of aging.

"A more recent study is based on people from Okinawa who live longer than any people on earth. The Okinawa Program combines elements of proper diet, physical exercise, a spontaneous—not rigid and hurried—view of time, social networks that act like healing webs, and a deep sense of spirituality into an entire way of life.[26]

"But for me, the most interesting study suggests that the challenge of growing older involves more than disease avoidance, physiological change, or lifestyle. David Curb claims that Effective

Aging means *compensating for* physiological changes and diseases. This view suggests that numerous non-physiological factors such as economic well-being, social support resources, availability and access to health services, and psychological well-being can and do influence lifestyle choices, which in turn affect whether we age effectively or not. Curb claims that people can compensate effectively through wisdom and experience for the declining physical skills that invariably accompany getting old."[27]

Bethany asks, "I wonder if there have been studies done on Effective Aging in lower socioeconomic groups?"

"I have some more detailed information that I can share with you after the session if you'd like, Bethany," Thomas says.

"Thanks," she responds and begins writing some of her ideas in her logbook.

Thomas moves on, "Using Curb's views as a backdrop for my own work has led me to some radical conclusions on Effective Aging. The *central claim* of this session is that the *specific factors* that compensate for physiological changes and diseases and lead to Effective Aging in a *specific individual* are actually diagnosed for that person by the Three Red Flags, especially the Unconscious's Perspective.

"Curb notes how most clinicians have had two seemingly similar patients with similar clinical problems who, for reasons unknown, experienced very different long-term outcomes in their functionality and well-being. My claim is that the difference between these patients may be the degree to which each one has answered the call to become themselves. On the one hand, people who are caught in the enormous power of driving forces of the Conscious Self and who lack the compensatory information that comes from the Unconscious Self, tend to live their lives in the throes of neurotic battles within their personality and consequently they are forced to endure *enormous stress*. On the other hand, people who answer the calling to become themselves and allow the Unconscious Self to guide them in the process live their lives differently and learn to use stress to their advantage. Whether or not we answer the calling to become ourselves may explain the clinical quandary mentioned above. My own sense is that the multiple factor model of the aging process mentioned by Curb might profitably add the factor of answering the calling to become ourselves to its matrix of the causes of aging.

"Effective Aging is more about creatively and dynamically experiencing and connecting to life than it is about how many *years* we have lived. This is why some people are rigid, narrow, and look *older* than people who are the very same age. In the first half of life, the Conscious Self must take control of situations and construct a life and a self. In the second half of life, we must answer the calling to discover who we are, which requires the Conscious Self to transition some of its control to the Emergent Self. The commitment to Effective Aging creates a deep and abiding appreciation for the mystery that lies in the biological-psychological interface: the mystery that we are biological-psychological beings that are inextricably bound within the human organism."

As Thomas pauses before wrapping up, Maggie turns to Lindsey and says loud enough for the entire group to hear, "I've always said there was a big difference between living long, and living well."

People nod in agreement as Thomas finishes, "I would like you to reflect on two things. First, 'How many of the elements of Effective Aging do I practice in my life?' Second, 'Are there specific compensatory factors that I am aware of that I need to include in my life?' Any questions? If not, then let's go diving."

As he got suited up, Thomas reflected on how paradoxically he had learned that while a careful and introspective analysis of oneself is *necessary*, it is not *sufficient* to enable us to continue on the path of discovering who we really are. Thomas had to learn to abandon his efforts to help himself and instead follow the calling, guidance, and teaching of the Unconscious Self. The path of self discovery is a process of continuous learning. Thomas had spent an enormous amount of time in the world of the Inner People and the unconscious and developed his skills in the Four Competencies. The exception was this Third Commitment. Especially now that he had become a father, the final step to experiencing true equanimity in his life and wholeness of personality would be to more fully keep his commitment to Effective Aging.

Once in the water, Thomas looked up at the surface and saw a few people still floating at about twenty feet. He assumed they were having trouble equalizing the pressure in their ears. He gave them the hand signal to ask if they were okay, and they pointed to their ears to tell him that they were having trouble getting down. This was the first trip where the entire group had dove this long without ear trouble. Most times, at least one or two people were forced to snorkel some of the dives toward the end of the week. The physics underwater is such that you get 50 percent of the full pressure of diving within the first thirty-three feet from the surface of the water, which is two atmospheres. Once you equalize the pressure in your ears to this depth, you feel almost no difference whether you are forty feet down or two hundred, which is why divers must always watch their depth. The underwater world is so unlike functioning on the surface, it's vital to stay present to the body and where you are in the water column.

~~~~~

By the time the bell rings for dinner at 7:00 P.M., people have to drag themselves to the table because they are all getting physically tired from the amount of diving they have been doing. Dan and James sit together and are wondering about other local dive sites. "Mike," James asks, "where are other good places to dive here in Indonesia?"

Mike gives it some thought and says, "Well not everywhere is as good as here, but I think that Wakatobi is a great place."

"Where is it?" Dan asks.

"It's a little island on the southeast tip of Sulawesi, just north of here. Another good place is Manado on the northern tip of Sulawesi."

Kirsten jumps in and says, "I'd go east to either Alor, which is just north of Timor, or to Sorong in Irian Jaya."

"Where's that?" James asks.

"You know how the front part of New Guinea looks like the mouth of an animal?" Kirsten gestures the shape with her hands. "Well, Papua, New Guinea is the back end with the tail, and Irian Jaya is the front end where the head is."

"Another place to go is Sipidan off the northeast coast of Borneo." Thomas adds, "It's a little island that you can walk around in about forty minutes, but it has some of the finest diving anywhere in the world." Mike and Kirsten nod their agreement as Thomas continues, "I'm actually offering a shore-based dive workshop there next year."

The conversation dies down, and Lindsey, James, Dan, and Maggie migrate to the upper deck to continue talking and relax before turning in. Everyone else heads straight to bed.

Day 5
EXPLORING THE SEA LIFE AROUND SANGEANG VOLCANO

THE DAY BEGINS

The *Explorer* has sailed all night and is anchored off of Sangeang Island. The twin peaks of the island are an active volcano that rise nearly ten thousand feet above the surface of the water. This is the same volcano that they saw days earlier when they did their very first dive of the trip off Satonda Island. This will be the last day of diving and there will only be workshop sessions for the first two dives, then the group will do a third dive, hoist the anchor and begin the eighteen-hour trip back to Benoa Harbor in Bali.

Over breakfast, Mike and Kirsten chat and answer questions about the dive sites at the foot of the volcano. It is a great place for what they call "muck" diving—digging through the black volcanic sand to find strange critters that can't be found anywhere else in the world.

SESSION 1: THE EMERGENT SELF

It's 8:05 A.M. and Mike rings the bell, and as people take their seats around the teaching table, Thomas stands at his flip chart simultaneously looking far away and deep within, absent to the world. A few seconds after everyone is seated, he breaks the silence.

"I want to talk about where we wind up when we decide to

answer the calling. If we commit time and the precious resource of psychological energy to this process, where *do* we wind up? What actually changes when we answer the calling in the second half of life? The *central claim* of this session is that the life-long journey of self discovery leads us to become the self that we were meant to be, an Emergent Self that rises from the collaboration and partnership of all parts of the personality. The result is that the *whole* personality is greater than the sum of the warring parts and that *greater* element is the Emergent Self.

"Perhaps I could use a metaphor to contrast a life lived with the Conscious Self in total control of the personality, and the life of a person who answers the calling to the process of discovering who they are. Let's do another thought experiment with this ship and a volcano."

Thomas points off the port side to the twin peaks of Sangeang rising almost two miles high above the surface of the ocean. "We already did a thought experiment about how a person who remains bound by the totalitarian control of the Conscious Self is like this ship, the reef, and the deep blue ocean. Do you remember Figure 3?" Thomas flips back to the diagram. "The entire scene is the personality, but the person is unaware of the life that exists beneath the surface of consciousness even though the vast majority of life comes from the reef and the deep blue ocean. All this person sees is what's above the surface of the water. More importantly, they are afraid to go down under the surface of consciousness for fear of what they might find. This person spends their entire life on the surface in the boat, and the life below goes on without them—it is objective, independent, and disconnected from the life of the person in the boat.

"But not all boats are the same, meaning not all Constructed Selves are the same. People who have lots of financial resources can build larger and more sea-worthy boats, and analogously, people who are born into certain families and have the resources of education, culture, and money can construct enormously robust Constructed Selves. Some people go through the storms of life in a twenty-foot tender like the ones we have been diving from. Other people have more resources so they build a hundred-foot ship like this one. And still others have the resources to construct enormous cruise ships like the *Sea Journey* that we saw anchored in Benoa harbor six days ago when we left Bali. For most people, how well you weather the storms of life is really about how big your boat is. Some Constructed Selves are almost invincible against even the biggest storms of life."

Dan comments, "How do people with the big boats in life ever come to realize that they need to change, especially if their boats are actually invincible? Why should they change?"

"I said these boats were *almost* invincible," Thomas responds. "One thing that all floating vessels have in common, regardless of their size, is they are constructed things, they are not natural things—they are man-made things. Like a jet that stays in the air by the force of its engines, vessels stay afloat by displacing the same water that constantly threatens to sink them. Once I was talking to a guy in a bar in the Florida Keys and told him that I owned some land on Plantation Key. The lot had a deeded slip in the marina and I was thinking of selling my house and buying a boat, putting it in the marina and living on it. He said, 'Boats are a black hole in the ocean into which you just keep pouring money.' That was probably the best advice I ever got."

Pointing up to the wheelhouse of the ship, Thomas says, "Ask our captain what he thinks. Keeping boats afloat is a never-ending process of repair and warding off the prospect of winding up on the bottom of the ocean.

"Regardless of the size and strength of your Conscious Self, it is man-made by you and requires an enormous amount of psychological maintenance to keep it afloat. You have to defend against slow leaks, or a catastrophe like hitting the invisible reef of the Inner People. Even a Conscious Self that is viewed as being unsinkable can go to the bottom of the deep blue sea if the right circumstances in life oppose it. The thing that is most disturbing and archetypal about the sinking of ships like the *Titanic* is that *there was no shore to go to*—they were in the middle of the deep blue sea of the crossing of life." Thomas points over the port side of the ship and says with a passion that radiates hope, "But islands do not sink like ships. Islands are not man-made objects. Islands are created naturally and the Emergent Self is like the island of that volcano.

"As we sail on the ocean of life, we begin to sense an enormous disturbance deep under the surface of the water of consciousness. The rumblings of the birth of the Emergent Self are like the lava flow deep beneath the surface of this water that resulted in Sangeang. Having risen high above the water, this magnificent island now sustains life, and is a place to land and find shelter during the storms of life. We can tell from the beauty of the reefs that the island of Sangeang is a magnet for life.

"When the calling comes and we refuse to listen, it is like trying to stop up the flow of lava deep under the water. Some people succeed more than others, but the lava cannot be fully stopped. If its flow is impeded and spreads out too much, it will never rise above the surface of the water of consciousness, and will never sustain life. In the same way, the Emergent Self rises out of the depths of our unconscious and becomes an *inner island* with white sandy beaches to which we can sail our ship, whatever its size. The partnership between the Unconscious Self and the Conscious Self is like a boat that can find harbor and a safe haven on the island, and still can sail the vessel to the surrounding reefs or out into the deep blue sea."

"Thomas," says James, "I still don't get why you call it the Emergent Self. How does it *emerge?*"

"Great question, James." Thomas nods his head affirmatively, "I was just coming to that. The Emergent Self rises out of the depths of the unconscious, but there is an even deeper meaning to the notion that it *emerges*. The notion of emergence often surfaces in discussions about the philosophical foundations of modern biology and physics. On one side of the discussion, physicists assert that all the theories of biology can, at least in principle, be reduced to theories in physics because all biological things are also physical things. But biologists insist that at a certain level of combinatorial complexity *unique* properties emerge— like life—that are not reducible to the physics of atomic structures. For example, I may have all the atoms that constitute my dog Tippy in a bucket, but in a very real sense, *I do not have Tippy*. I might be able to reduce the sound of Vivaldi's *The Four Seasons* into its constituent frequencies, but I no longer have Vivaldi. Novel, unique, animated, thinking, complex, elegant, philosophically profound, psychological properties *do emerge* at higher levels of combinatorial complexity, and they *are not* directly reducible to fundamental constituents.

"More importantly, these emergent properties are *real* in the sense that they make a physical difference in the world. Tippy's atoms in a bucket cannot play with me, steal food from the kitchen counter, bark at me, or demand that I give him his dinner and then take him for a walk. Tippy can, and does, do all of these very real things every day. The commonsense way of expressing the principle of emergence is that *the whole is greater than the sum of the parts*. The Emergent Self is a property of the wholeness of the human personality, that is *not directly reducible* to the constituent psychic elements we have been discussing up until now. It is an emergent property of the human personality that *does not exist* when the personality is under siege with inner civil war."

"I've often found that when I'm working with a team that is really clicking together well," said Lindsey, "a spirit of productivity and cooperation emerges that really is greater than the sum of the parts of the individual people."

"Yeah," James proffers, "it's like that in sports too, with winning teams." Various members of the group nod in agreement.

Thomas is pleased that the group is really diving into the material, and forges ahead. "We discover that the Unconscious Self really wants to collaborate in the process of organizing, harmonizing, and unifying all of the complexes in the human personality. When we first answer the calling, the Conscious Self is terrified because it experiences the inner wilderness as its own *death*. But once the Conscious Self submits to numerous cycles of growth, it experiences a kind of *rebirth* that is archetypal in nature. As the Conscious Self comes to trust that psychological life follows what appears to be psychological death, it increasingly gives up its repressive stranglehold on consciousness. In an unexpected way, the Conscious Self learns that the Unconscious Self is actually collaborating with it for the mutual benefit of the entire personality.[28]

"The Unconscious Self *counteracts* the natural tendency toward entropy within the personality and increasingly mediates between the opposing forces of the Triangle of Duplicity and the Inner People, all of whom are determined to hoard as much psychological energy and facility time as possible. The end result is that the Unconscious Self draws the Triangle of Duplicity, the Inner People, and the archetypes to itself so as to unite the entire human personality."

Thomas crosses to his flip chart and turns the page. "The collaboration between all the complexes results in a major shift in the overall control of the human personality from the Conscious Self who was the *center of consciousness*, to the Emergent Self who becomes the *center of the personality*. This is shown in Figure 10.

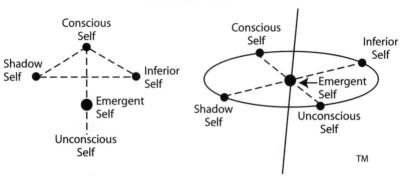

Figure 10

INNER GYROSCOPIC
EMERGENT SELF

"We experience this shift to a mid-point as an Inner Gyroscopic Sense of Orientation along the Axis of Self. The Emergent Self and the totality of our personality and our inner and outer lives have a new *virtual center* that unifies them and makes them much more difficult to perturb. We realize that we have a deep, hidden place of safety and guidance that will help us lead our lives."

"Thomas!" Bethany blurts out, almost stopping him in mid-sentence. "Can I share an insight that I just had?"

"Sure, go for it." Thomas smiles.

"For the first part of the dive workshop, I couldn't connect experientially to the inner sense of guidance you talked about, and I couldn't find a solution that took me beyond this impasse. As you were talking a minute ago, the idea that the Unconscious Self would actually lead me if I just follow the Three Red Flags *clicked* in my head. I have more than enough examples of Unintended Consequences and Defense Mechanisms in my life, so if they really are inner mooring balls then *they* become the concrete examples of the true inner guidance that I've been looking for."

"Yes, you've got it." Thomas nods in agreement, and Bethany continues. "The fact that I can experientially trust this much of what you're saying starts to feel like a foundation that I can build on. I'm still having a difficult time experiencing the Inner Gyroscopic Sense of Orientation, but I'm powerfully drawn to the visual image of Figure 10, and I want to begin to sense the place of inner peace, tranquility, and orientation that you have been talking about."

Bethany will have to come to terms with the distinction described early on in the workshop, which called her to abandon her search for ultimate "truth" and absolute certainty and instead cling to the notion of reliability as the best that life has to offer. Despite the mirage of absolute certainty that her ultra-fundamentalist faith in God tried to provide, she always feels lost in a constantly moving inner and outer sea of justifications and rationalizations that she suspects cannot really support their claims. Learning to experience the inner guidance and teaching of the Unconscious Self may actually strengthen her faith in God, by not placing such rigid and legalistic demands on how she views herself, other people, and the world around her.

Thomas continues, "Following the guidance of the Unconscious Self, who teaches us how to develop increasing skill in the Four Competencies and the Three Commitments, is sufficient to answer the calling to discover who you are. But for those of you who are interested in *accelerating* this process, here are five additional ways you can do this.

"First, learn about the Enneagram and use it as a diagnostic tool to discover the inner conflict within the Triangle of Duplicity. Take the Enneagram type numbers that you filled in for Figure 4 and read and reflect on the degree to which these three sets of characteristics actually describe and predict the conflict in the Triangle of Duplicity in your life. Don Richard Riso gives extensive empirical descriptions of the behavior, fears, motivations, and emotional patterns of the nine personality types. The value of the Riso-Hudson Enneagram is that even people with little or no experience with, or aptitude for, introspection and self-exploration can gain enormous insights into themselves by reading the description of their type. Consequently, our Enneagram type allows us to peer into the very deepest and most obscure empirical aspects of the values, beliefs, and personality traits of the Conscious Self and the Inner People. When the Conscious Self, the Emergent Self, and the Unconscious Self are all aligned along the Axis of Self, this builds a Basic Trust within the total personality that all of the complexes will survive. We experience this kind of deep, inner alignment in all aspects of our everyday life."

Thomas takes a step away from his flip chart, turns, faces the group and says, "But the Enneagram must be used with caution. Although it is an incredibly powerful *shortcut* to mapping out the deeper elements of the Conscious Self and the Triangle of Duplicity, this tool can fall into the wrong psychological hands. In much the same way the Conscious Self can incorporate insights from therapy, self-help books, et cetera, into its arsenal of defenses, the Enneagram can become a powerful exercise in *perpetuating* the inner civil war. In other words, if we don't view the human personality as a set of fragmented psychological complexes that are objective to one's Enneagram type, we remain in the realm of *self* help. This can never lead to the kind of deep personal change that is required to answer the calling of discovering who we are."

"I realize now," Nikki interjects, "that this is part of the reason that I came to a standstill in my psychological growth using the Enneagram."

Thomas grins, "I know other people who have hit the same type of brick wall of psychological growth using the Enneagram improperly. Now to continue, the second way to accelerate the process of discovering who we are is to find experiences that put you into the spectator role like this workshop—movies, plays, books, people-watching or any other situation—that allows you to view yourself and the people in your life from a distance. You can use these situations to gain perspective about yourself that you can have in no other way.

"Third, keep a journal that records the twists and turns of the *labyrinth* of discovering who you are. The journal should mirror the structure of the Four Competencies so that it becomes a *vessel* into which you pour the contents of your life experiences. Ask the Conscious Self to step aside as you write in the journal and your entries will often articulate the perspective of the Inner People and the Unconscious Self. When you follow the calling, guiding, and teaching of the Unconscious Self as an *inner diver*, you will be led to explore your relationships, memories, professional life, and myriad other issues identified by the Three Red Flags. The inner exploration of the set of circumstances, people and issues that cluster around each Red Flag and the synthesis of opposing forces within you become a kind of *mini process* of psychological growth within the *life-long process* of discovering who you are. While these mini processes may seem random and unrelated, codifying your life experiences over time in a journal will reveal the cumulative pattern of your life's calling like a multiplicity of streams that feed into the deep underground river of your life. The hidden pattern of your calling can only be seen from a distance and will emerge over time."

Thomas flips back through the pages of his flip chart until he finds Figure 1 and continues. "I try to view the process of self discovery from a distance once a year by having a personal retreat during which I reflect on the contents of my journal, make course corrections, and set goals that I want to accomplish in the areas shown here in Figure 1. When you use your journal as the basis of an annual retreat, it will act as a Facilitator of Change because it mirrors back to you crucial aspects of the journey toward wholeness, including the nature and characteristics of your Emergent Self."

The people sitting around the wooden teaching table are writing furiously in the logbook they received on the first day of the dive workshop. The insights and issues they have logged over the course of the six days *have become* the kind of journal that Thomas is talking about. Thomas takes a step away from his flip chart and continues.

"Fourth, you can accelerate the process of discovering who you are and bring an increased level of accountability to keeping your journal by finding a Personal Coach to work with. People seek out a Personal Coach when they are: making major life decisions, changing jobs or careers, experiencing interpersonal conflict in their business or personal life, trying to harness the power of their creativity, or feeling stuck and unmotivated about their relationships or professional life. A Personal Coach helps you *link* the decisions and issues that you face on the surface of your life with the deep longing, which most people have, to find your destiny—your special calling in life.

"A Personal Coach is someone who has answered the calling to discover who they are and who becomes a Facilitator of Change in your personal or professional life. There are two main requirements to look for when choosing a Personal Coach. First, can the tools they use actually ignite deep, profound, sustainable personal change, or are they quick-fix, band-aid approaches that require discipline, trying harder, and thinking positively. Second, are they actively involved in walking the path of the calling to self-discovery? A Personal Coach is like an *inner dive master* who buddies up with you, and helps facilitate the process of *inner diving*—someone who helps you navigate important changes and transitions.

"A Personal Coach *models* the process of discovering who you are and can help you listen for the deep, often quiet, inner flow of the river of destiny that comes from the Unconscious Self. They also hold you accountable for acting on the knowledge that you gain from the coaching process and help you define an individual path for moving forward in life. A partnership with a Personal Coach is different from the relationship of a client to a therapist or analyst. A coaching partnership assumes that the person being coached is psychologically healthy and not in an on-going, neurotic crisis that requires professional psychological intervention. Personal Coaching is about discovering who you really are and what your destiny is in life. It is not a *substitute* for professional psychological treatment."

Thomas walks to the portion of the teaching table where Lindsey is sitting and says, "The fifth way to accelerate your journey of self-discovery is to enter the formal process of Jungian analysis with an analyst. Many people believe that the various types of professional psychologists and psychiatrists are all the same, but they are not. There is a critical difference between traditional psychotherapy and the analytical psychology of Carl Jung. Most psychotherapy is designed as intervention and treatment that helps people deal with the emotions and behaviors that cause on-going, neurotic crisis in relationships and interactions with the world. While approaches to psychotherapy vary widely, many of them involve the process of raising consciousness about the blind spots and defense mechanisms that protect unhealthy psychological and behavioral routines. A psychotherapist is a Facilitator of Change because they help to raise a client's consciousness by mirroring unhealthy routines back to them until the person can see the causes of their problems for themselves. The ultimate goal of a therapist should be to get a client to the point where *they can facilitate their own process*—and be their own therapist and Facilitator of Change."

Thomas begins pacing in front of the teaching table with visible intensity as he presses on. "We begin to see the differences between psychotherapy and analysis when we discuss the issue of how the therapist and client decide what to discuss during the therapeutic session. Or more pointedly, when we ask the question, 'what is it that guides the overall direction of the therapeutic process?' Many times, a therapist's opening chitchat of, 'So how's your week been?' leads to topics of immediate concern to the client, but often these 'crisis' issues are of little value to obtaining deep personal change.

"One difference between analysis and psychotherapy is that the direction of analysis is led by the calling, guiding, and teaching functions of the Unconscious Self through the Three Red Flags, not by the therapist or analyst. Second, whereas most therapeutic approaches assume a single unified sense of self, the model of personality we have been discussing views the Inner People, Unconscious Self, and the archetypes of the collective unconscious as being independent of, and objective to, the Conscious Self. This distinction becomes crucial when the analysand (client) experiences the powerful and sometimes bizarre emotions of the Inner People and the archetypes *as their own.*

"Another difference is that in analysis the analyst and the analysand consciously allow the calling, guiding, and teaching roles of the Unconscious Self to be externalized and projected onto the arena of the analytical relationship. This process of focusing on the Unconscious's Perspective that is revealed through the Three Red Flags *purposely introduces* psychological imbalance into the psyche of the analysand—an imbalance that the analyst helps to contain and interpret. Focusing on the Unconscious's Perspective begins to *dissolve* the pretenses and facades that the Conscious Self has spent a lifetime *protecting.* Together, the analyst and the analysand *explore* the shadowy and undeveloped complexes and archetypes in the personality as they are revealed by the Unconscious's Perspective. As with psychotherapy, the ultimate goal of analysis is for the analyst to work themselves out of a job—to teach the analysand to facilitate their own process of self-discovery."

"Whether you choose to accelerate the process or not," Thomas again points to Figure 10, "the partnership along the Axis of Self motivates us to live out of the Basic Trust that all complexes of our personality will survive. This produces a deep and abiding sense of hope about ourselves, other people, life, and the prospects for finding our destiny. We read about it in the lives of people like Gandhi, Patton, and Martin Luther King. Many people hunger and thirst to experience the calling in their lives, that's why people who have answered the calling touch something deep within us.

"I'd like you to reflect on two things during the next dive." Thomas pauses, grabs his glass of water and wets his parched throat. "First, reflect on the thought experiment of the ship and the island. Second, ask yourself, 'What things can I do to accelerate the process of answering my own calling?' Are there any questions?"

Bethany raises her hand. "What does this inner shift to the Emergent Self feel like experientially? How do you know it when you see it?"

"Look for the Inner Gyroscopic Sense of Orientation," Thomas answers. "Gyroscopes are mounted inside spaceships and you can turn a ship upside down or in any direction, but the gyroscope doesn't lose its orientation—that's why they use them in space. Look at the drawing in Figure 10, close your eyes, and try to imagine that that gyroscope has emerged from deep within you. When times get hard in life, look inwardly for that gyroscope to find your *center*, the place of inner orientation. When you have this Inner Gyroscopic Sense of Orientation, the ups and downs of life are still real, but they do not cause you to lose your psychological orientation in life.

"Another way to think about it, where you formerly felt you were adrift at sea in the ship of your Conscious Self—whatever its size— toughing out the storms of life, the Emergent Self rises from within the abyss of the depths of the blue sea. Metaphorically, you will begin to feel like your feet have found, and can trust, a new kind of inner solid ground. When the Emergent Self begins to make its presence known, it is like the emergence of an inner island in the midst of the ocean of your unconscious."

The distinction between *having* a destiny and *creating* one breaks into Nikki's consciousness with the force and power of the ocean. She has always had to take her life into her own hands by planning her life out and then brute-forcing people, situations, and all of life into conforming to her plans—do-want, push-control. She had created her own destiny, but what if she really *has* a destiny independent of her efforts and plans? What if staying present to the calling, guiding, teaching presence of the Unconscious Self will reveal that destiny, and all she has to do is to let it unfold moment by moment? This shift in focus from creating a destiny to having one and letting it unfold will force her to wait in the existential now and swear off the intoxicating effects of staying in motion. The increasing presence of the Emergent Self in her life holds the promise and the hope of new inner life that will spring from the barren inner wilderness she has known from childhood. The inner desert of dry bones will live again, and she will find a life where she lives soberly in the present moment, in the existential now of life.

Thomas sees Nikki writing furiously in her logbook, and begins to pace as he continues, "The outcome of the process of discovering who you are is not just a psychological thing. The existence and characteristics of the Emergent Self is fully anchored to the pedestrian aspects of everyday life in the Three Commitments. We see it in how we make a difference in life with projects we undertake either at work or at home. We see it in our relationships with family, friends, neighbors, working associates—our portfolio begins to be different. We see it in how we treat the totality of our body and mind through Effective Aging. Any other comments? If not, let's go diving."

～～～～

James was amazed at the bubbles rising out of the dark volcanic sand. He pushed his hand about six inches beneath the surface and he could feel the heat of the volcano emanating in the bubbles that covered the sea floor. The underwater topography was unusual here, with long stretches of barren sand emanating bubbles, interspersed with pinnacles of coral that were even more colorful against the underwater background of the black volcanic sand. The social structure of the group had gone from individual teams of "buddies" to almost more of a group dive where people dove with and watched out for each other, without getting in other people's dive space.

The thing about diving is that even if you're with a group, you still have the solitude of your own psychological space once you are under the water. Dan tried to visualize the lava thousands of feet below the sandy surface, the way the volcano rose from nothing, the life that emerged on the reef, and he tried to relate this to his own experiences and the change he was hoping to make after the workshop.

SESSION 2: SOME FINAL THOUGHTS

It's 11:00 A.M. when Thomas rings the bell, then he walks to his flip chart and chats with Bethany and Lindsey while the others are getting seated. Once everyone is in their places, he begins, "I want to talk about the life-long process of answering the calling in more concrete terms to prepare you as you head home to your life, work, and families. I was once on a dive trip on the Great Barrier Reef, and one of the crew, who knew a lot about marine life, would always say, 'The more you know, the more you see.' I never forgot that. It's easy to get overwhelmed by the sheer number of types of coral and fish here in Indonesia. But if you take the time to learn about the different types of sea life, that increased knowledge pays big dividends. Then when you dive a site like Cannibal Rock multiple times and begin to tease apart the difference between the hundreds of kinds of hard and soft coral, identify rare fish and mollusks that can be seen nowhere else in the world, each dive seems different. The more you know, the more you see.

"Psychological growth is the same way: the more you know, the more you see, but knowing and seeing is a continuous process that spirals us to higher and higher levels of psychological health and maturity." Thomas turns the page on his flip chart, points to a diagram, "Figure 11 shows the four phases of psychological growth that were originated by William Howell.[29] Whether it is a problematic relationship or some specific issue in life, we begin in the first phase of *Unconscious Incompetence*, where we have issues and problems that press upon us in day-to-day life, but are unaware that there is even a problem.

Figure 11
THE CYCLE OF CONTINUOUS PSYCHOLOGICAL GROWTH

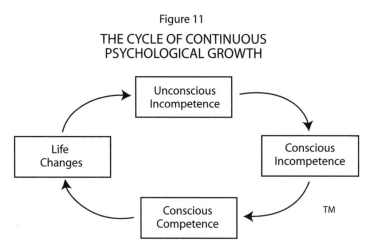

"In the second phase of *Conscious Incompetence*, the Three Red Flags confront us with wave after wave of empirical evidence that forces us to admit that we are unable to solve the problems of life without the calling, guiding, and teaching roles of the Unconscious Self. Once the opposing forces in the personality are synthesized and the formerly fixated energy is freed-up and channeled into making and keeping the Three Commitments, we move into the final phase of *Conscious Competence*. This is the stage of life where we feel good about our level of psychological health, and how we're handling the people and situations in our lives. Eventually, that competency becomes a habit that falls below the level of consciousness and becomes tacit knowledge that we use on automatic pilot. Then, *Life Changes*. New problems emerge in life that we may or may not be aware of, and we unknowingly migrate back into the phase of Unconscious Incompetence and begin the cycle again at the bidding of the Unconscious Self. But this time we know more about the depths of our personality and life, and consequently we see more ways to approach the new issues that face us. That's why the very First Competency that the Unconscious Self teaches us is new insight into the totality of the human personality."

Thomas takes slow, careful steps in front of his flip chart as he speaks. "If the dive workshop has changed your paradigm and the way you view yourself, it will probably also change the way you view other people and the world around you. Because you know more, you will see more. You will see the world differently."

Thomas stops and faces the group directly, "I want to talk about three tangible differences that you will see in your lives as you continue along the path of discovering who you really are.

"First, as you gain increased knowledge about the totality of the human personality you will be increasingly *motivated by the Basic Trust* that all aspects of your personality will survive rather than being *driven by the Basic Fear* of biological and psychological survival.

"Second, as you stop identifying with the Conscious Self, and the Inner People and the conflict in the Triangle of Duplicity subsides, you will begin to experience the presence of the Emergent Self for the very first time. You will become more aware of the Inner Gyroscopic Sense of Orientation as the whole of your personality becomes greater than the sum of the warring parts.

"Third, you will begin to discover your destiny in the sense that you both *have* a destiny, and you must *create* your own destiny. Your destiny will be your individual path in life that you must walk in answer to the archetypal pattern of existential questions that are presented to you by life."

"I've heard the word destiny all my life, but I have never heard it described so succinctly—it's just my individual path to the big questions in life," Dan says in amazement. Some of the other members of the group mumble their agreement.

Wrapping up the workshop, Thomas says, "And last, as you head home, I want to remind you about three final things. First, if you travel back to work, friends, and family and walk the path of self discovery and experience deep personal change, but no one else mirrors that back to you, you are the final judge.

"Second, the process of discovering who you are is objective and independent of the material presented during the dive workshop." Thomas holds up the book about marine life that people have been studying all week, and moves to the railing of the ship. "The process of discovering who you are is a natural, biological-psychological process— just like the life on the reef exists independent of this book about marine life. The calling of the Unconscious Self makes its presence known to all people, of all ages, in all places of the world regardless of what people call it.

"Third, during the dive workshop I have tried to function like an *inner dive master* who led you into the deep places below the surface of your consciousness. I have also tried to be a Facilitator of Change by holding up a mirror of what I see in you, in the hopes that you will begin to see it in yourself. As you leave the boat, you must increasingly experience the calling, guidance, and teaching of the Unconscious Self for yourself—it will become your inner dive master. The Unconscious Self is the one who knows the inner reefs, who knows the way back to the boat of consciousness, who knows how to read the currents of life, and the one who will teach you a healthy fear of the depths of the unconscious. Are there any questions? Okay," Thomas says with a wide smile on his face, "for the *last time*, let's go diving!"

∿∿∿∿∿

The tenders reached the dive site in no time, and the two groups of divers quickly dropped into the water. As Dan began to relax and enjoy the solitude of the underwater world, he became more and more convinced that he needed the kind of deep personal change that Thomas was talking about. A large part of this change would be for him to gain skill in the Four Competencies and to make and keep the Three Commitments. Dan needed change that was real, change that made a physical difference in the world. Real change would allow Dan to tease apart the distinction between the many times he had talked about changing, made promises to change, intended to change, hoped he could change, or kept explaining to Susan how he was really working on change. Whatever happened on this journey of self-discovery, the change he had already felt happening within him had to be cashed out, concretized, and instantiated in the world, or else his talk and all the insights he gained during the dive workshop would not add up to real change.

The bell rings at 3:00 P.M., but oddly, it is not calling them to gather around the great wooden teaching table—instead it is time for the last dive of the trip. Mike and Kirsten have picked a relaxing dive site on a part of the reef that teems with Indonesian marine life. The dive crew wants the group's last dive to be a memorable one.

An hour later when they are back on *Explorer*, people are sharing stories about the animals and coral they saw, rinsing off their dive gear in the two large rinse tanks on the main deck, and hanging it up to dry. The ship is filled with activity. Part of the crew hauls the tenders up onto the main boat, while others raise the anchor and still others begin hoisting the deep blue sails of *Explorer* to begin the journey back to Bali.

Dan is one of the first people to finish rinsing his gear, so out of habit he grabs his usual chair at the teaching table and stares out over the railing across the sea. Prior to coming on the trip, Dan had somehow lost his way in life, but only now does he realize this. How will he apply what he has learned in the workshop at home with Susan and Carol? Will the change that has begun on this trip stand the test of time in the mundane, pedestrian realities of life? How can he apply what he has learned back at the office? Even on casual reflection he knows that people put up with him and his outbursts because they are trapped in a world where they need their job and can't just walk away from it. They just suck it in and absorb it like a sponge.

Dan has begun to feel a whole new sense of connection with Cindy, knowing she has been on this same trip. In some way, Cindy reminds him of Thomas. Maybe they are the same Enneagram type. Dan has still not spoken with Thomas privately about his dream, and he knows he will need additional help if he is really going to stay the course of the process of discovery. Maybe Thomas can help sort things out with his company?

Dan wanders upstairs and sits up on the back upper deck. This is the place people go when they want to get some space and be alone. The sky is the brightest blue he can ever remember, and he feels free, maybe for the first time in his life. In silence he stares at the wake of the *Explorer* that looks like two white lines extending far off the back of the ship, then disappearing into the deep blue sea off on the horizon. With each second that he watches the ship's wake, he feels he is moving further and further in time and space from the places that he first got the insights that have helped him to know himself in a new and different way. Dan now feels confident that change is a real possibility for him. He believes that he is ready to answer the calling in this, the second half of life. As the glorious Indonesian sun looks like it's about to plunge into the ocean, Dan says to himself with a smile, "And, there's no time like the present to begin *diving in*."

Epilogue (One Year Later)

RICK FLOWTON'S father-in-law, Frank, meets him at the airport on his return from the dive workshop and Frank is heartened when he sees how excited Rick is about the prospect of change in his life. But within a few weeks Frank knows that whatever change happened was short-term. Within a few months of Rick's return, Frank hires someone to run the northern location and brings Rick back to the main office as his special assistant. He tries to find useful things for Rick to do, but by-and-large, Rick is warehoused at a high salary, just like Joanne had predicted. Frank's focus on the bottom-line makes carrying Rick difficult. But Frank is still torn, just as he was before Rick went to the dive workshop. He knows that if he fires Rick, his daughter and grandchildren will suffer, possibly lose their house, and have to move back in with him, which he finds even more intolerable than just paying Rick a salary for doing nothing. Unfortunately, this solution further supports Rick's philosophy that things will work out if he just goes with the flow.

By all measures **Lindsey Barker** is a psychologically "normal" person, but after returning from the dive workshop she wants to build her sense of who she is on a complete understanding of all parts of her personality, rather than just a façade of being a giving servant to everyone. She continues to use the principles she learned in the dive workshop and begins the process of analysis with a Jungian analyst, with the goal of exploring the hidden parts of her personality. She experiences deep, profound, sustainable change in her life—change that begins to permeate into all of her relationships. People at the office sense the difference in her because she is more transparent, open and honest about her desire to be in charge. Eventually, even her former detractors support Mario's decision to reorganize and promote her to Vice President over the administrative side of the company. More importantly, she focuses on the Second Commitment of making a difference in life and increasingly channels her time and psychological energy into her creative abilities and finding an identity for herself outside her relationships.

The battle with environmentalists has escalated while **Maggie Spinner** was at the dive workshop. Her boss, J.R., is shocked when she comes into his office on the Monday of her return and confronts him about what she knows and threatens to turn the company in to the authorities and the local press. He promises to cease the poisonous discharge immediately, and then offers Maggie an enormous separation package if she will leave the company and agree not to reveal what she knows. Maggie turns down what she views as hush money, leaves the company, and decides to take some time to clear her head. She spends more and more time in Winter Park with Troy. He is good for her and they begin to talk about making their relationship more permanent. Maggie decides to start a marketing and advertising agency in Boulder and calls it the Spinner Group. By the end of the year, she builds an impressive client portfolio and is making a difference in the success of their businesses. Her daughter, Rena, graduates from Colorado College with a degree in business and marketing and joins the new company. Eventually, Rena will open a branch office of the Spinner Group in Colorado Springs.

Thomas Rose headed home to Kona on the Big Island of Hawaii to be with his wife, Grace, and their son, Mark. The most powerful lesson Thomas has learned during the dive workshops is that he needs to renew his commitment to Effective Aging. Within a few months, he is back to running five times a week and has lost twenty-five pounds. Exercise and proper diet does even more for Thomas's head than for his body. Thomas feels a renewed sense of creativity and psychological energy to continue his existing workshops and to focus on developing new workshops.

Joel Booker's workload only increases when he returns from the dive workshop and his relationship with his wife Pat becomes increasingly distant and strained. Joel always apologizes when his wife confronts him about the way he treats her, and he appears to go along with what she says, but secretly he has no intention of changing. At the laboratory, a computer-monitoring system installed by the Computing Division reveals that Joel has been spending enormous amounts of time visiting pornographic Web sites on government time, including child pornography. By this time, Pat is in the process of divorcing him and is trying to get sole custody of his daughter, Sarah, partly on the basis of his interest in child pornography and some accusations she makes against Joel about his behavior with Sarah.

Bethany Wringer decides to begin to take control of her life away from her ultra-fundamentalist parents. Within a year, she marries Matt, becomes a member of the Lutheran church he attends, and transfers Samuel to her new church's daycare, which is much better staffed. This makes her parents furious and they continually harp on her with a kind of self-righteous indignation. Matt is the general manager at a local grocery store, and becomes a good stepfather to Samuel and they are making plans to have another child. Formerly, Bethany's ultra-fundamentalist religion projected the mirage of absolute certainty, but she begins to discover the guidance of the Unconscious Self and follows it. This produces a deep and abiding sense of inner reliability and an Inner Gyroscopic Sense of Orientation about life. Slowly, she abandons the rigid, legalistic, Victorian view of herself and life, and even the way she dresses changes to reflect that.

Nikki Salem decides to take a job as director of production for the home office of the cosmetic company she works for so she can stop traveling so much. She continuously confronts her obsession with staying in constant motion, and is genuinely concerned with discovering how she can leave a legacy in life. She begins to learn to stop and seek the inner calling, guidance, and teaching of her Unconscious Self, and finds that life unfolds for her naturally. Within six months after the dive workshop, she has met a guy named Conner. As she learns to give of herself, time, money, communication, and other resources in life that she used to fear might be taken from her, she begins to build a long-term relationship and sees new life emerge from the inner wilderness of her formerly barren soul.

James Tuffs continues to grow his law practice and he becomes more and more involved in the Episcopal Church he attends in Breckenridge. The inner path and calling that he sensed even prior to attending the dive workshop begins to lead him into the process of ministerial discernment and to becoming a priest. In a conversation with the Bishop of Colorado, James discovers that he can continue to support his family with his law practice, and take a kind of home study program that will train him for the priesthood. James has a vision to start a small mission church in the town of Fairplay, six miles south of his home, and he does just that. Once he is ordained, he becomes the part-time priest of that parish. The church grows under James's leadership and it becomes a place of sanctuary and spiritual renewal for all who attend.

Dan Wright decides to focus on two priorities after returning from the dive workshop. The first is his relationship with his wife, Susan, and his daughter, Carol. The Enneagram helps Dan to realize that his wife has an enormous self-esteem problem and feels like nobody special. As he focuses on her and her needs, and puts aside his obsession with always being right, slowly the relationship heals and eventually a renewed sense of love emerges between them.

Dan's second focus is to develop a succession plan for SciTech. Despite the improvement in his relationship with his daughter, Carol, she does not want to replace Dan as the President of SciTech. Surprisingly, Cindy Reeder agrees to take over the presidency within a year, on the condition that Dan will hire a Chief Operating Officer to run the day-to-day affairs of the company. She also asks Dan to form a Board of Directors that he will chair, so he can provide periodic input to Cindy and the company. Both Dan and Cindy stay in touch with Thomas, who agrees to help them with the process of transitioning the presidency from Dan to Cindy.

BRIEF SUMMARY OF ENNEAGRAM TYPES

The characters in this book are based on the nine personality types of a personality typology called the Enneagram. The Enneagram not only describes and predicts how we behave, it also describes many of the deeper motivations of human behavior. Perhaps the most accessible treatment of the Enneagram is the work of Don Richard Riso and Russ Hudson. The Enneagram descriptions below are based on Riso-Hudson's extensive discussion of each Enneagram type in their books, *Personality Types* and *The Wisdom of the Enneagram*.[30] The reader can use the descriptions below as a quick reference when reading through the book, or obtain more detailed descriptions from the Riso-Hudson books.

Figure 12

DIVING IN ENNEAGRAM TYPES

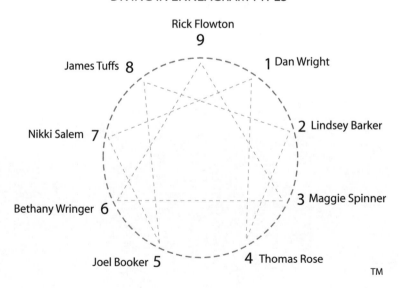

Type One

People who are principled, orderly, self-controlled, perfectionistic, and self-righteous. "They are teachers, crusaders, and advocates for change: always striving to improve things, but afraid to make a mistake."[31]

Type Two

People who are caring, interpersonal, empathic, sincere, and warm-hearted. "They are friendly, generous, and self-sacrificing, but can also be sentimental, flattering, and people-pleasing."[32]

Type Three

People who are adaptable, success-oriented, self-assured, attractive, and charming. "Ambitious, competent, and energetic, they can also be status-conscious and highly driven for advancement."[33]

Type Four

People who are introspective, romantic, self-aware, sensitive, and reserved. "They are emotionally honest, creative, and personal, but can also be moody and self-conscious."[34]

Type Five

People who are perceptive, intellectually alert, insightful, and curious. "They are able to concentrate and focus on developing complex ideas and skills... they can also become preoccupied with their thoughts and imaginary constructs."[35]

Type Six

People who are committed, security-oriented, reliable, hardworking, responsible and trustworthy. "Excellent 'troubleshooters,' they foresee problems and foster cooperation, but can also become defensive, evasive, and anxious—running on stress while complaining about it."[36]

Type Seven

People who are busy, productive, playful, high-spirited, and practical. "They can also misapply their many talents, becoming over-extended, scattered, and undisciplined."[37]

Type Eight

People who are powerful, aggressive, self-confident, strong, and assertive. "Protective, resourceful, straight-talking, and decisive, but can also be ego-centric and domineering."[38]

Type Nine

People who are easy-going, self-effacing, accepting, trusting, and stable. "They are usually creative, optimistic, and supportive, but can also be too willing to go along with others to keep the peace."[39]

ENDNOTES

1   For a detailed discussion of the Nine Enneagram Types see Don Richard Riso with Russ Hudson, *Personality Types: Using the Enneagram for Self Discovery*, (New York: Houghton Mifflin Company, 1996).

2   An on-line version of the Riso Hudson Enneagram Type Indicator (RHETI), or hard copies, can be obtained from the Enneagram Institute's Web site—www.enneagraminstitute.com.

3   See the description of the Type One on the RHETI and the detailed discussion in, Riso, *Personality Types*, pp. 376–409.

4   See the description of the Type Two on the RHETI and the detailed discussion in, Riso, *Personality Types*, pp. 59–94.

5   See the description of the Type Three on the RHETI and the detailed discussion in, Riso, *Personality Types*, pp. 95–133.

6   See the description of the Type Eight on the RHETI and the detailed discussion in, Riso, *Personality Types*, pp. 297–337.

7   See the description of the Type Nine on the RHETI and the detailed discussion in, Riso, *Personality Types*, pp. 338–375.

8   See the description of the Type Seven on the RHETI and the detailed discussion in, Riso, *Personality Types*, pp. 259–296.

9   Clarisa Pinkola Estes, *Women Who Run with the Wolves: Myths and Stories of the Wild Woman Archetype*, (New York: Ballantine Books, 1995), p. 53.

10   See the description of the Type Six on the RHETI and the detailed discussion in, Riso, *Personality Types*, pp. 216–258.

11   See the description of the Type Four on the RHETI and the detailed discussion in, Riso, *Personality Types*, pp. 134–172.

12   See the description of the Type Five on the RHETI and the detailed discussion in, Riso, *Personality Types*, pp. 173–215.

13   Abraham Maslow, *Toward a Psychology of Being*, 3rd ed., (New York: John Wiley & Sons, 1999), p. 27 ff.

14   Don Richard Riso and Russ Hudson, *The Wisdom of the Enneagram: The Complete Guide to Psychological and Spiritual Growth for the Nine Personality Types*, (New York: Bantam Books, 1999), and Sandra Maitri, *The Spiritual Dimension of the Enneagram: Nine Faces of the Soul*, (New York: Jeremy P. Tarcher, Putnam, 2000).

15   Carl G. Jung, "The Psychogenesis of Mental Disease," Volume 3 in *The Collected Works of C.G. Jung*, (Princeton, NJ: Princeton University Press, 1976), par. 525, p. 242.

16   Carl R. Rogers, "Barriers and Gateways to Communication," in the *Harvard Business Review*, July-August 1952, Number 52408, and Carl R. Rogers, *On Becoming a Person: A Therapist's View of Psychotherapy* (Boston: Houghton Mifflin Company, 1961), p. 330.

17   J.K. Rowling, *Harry Potter and the Philosopher's Stone*, (London: Bloomsbury, 1997), p. 204 ff, and J.R.R. Tolkien, *The Lord of the Rings: The Fellowship of the Ring*, (London: Collins, 1991).

18   See Chris Argyris, Robert Putnam, Diana McLaim Smith, *Action Science: Concepts, Methods, and Skills for Research and Intervention*, (San Francisco: Jossey-Bass Publishers, 1985).

19   Estes, *Women Who Run with the Wolves*, p. 44.

20   Estes, *Women Who Run with the Wolves*, p. 52.

21   Graham Wallas, *The Art of Thought*, (London: Jonathan Cape, 1926).

22   Rollo May, *The Courage to Create*, (New York: W.W. Norton & Company Inc., 1975), pp. 19 and 24.

23   Hans Selye, *Stress without Distress*, (New York: J.B. Lippincott Company, 1974), p. 38 and 39.

24   John W. Rowe and Robert L. Kahn, *Successful Aging*, (New York: Pantheon Books, 1998), pp. 38–39.

25   Peter J. D'Adamo, *Live Right for Your Blood Type: The Individualized Prescription for Maximizing Health, Metabolism, and Vitality in Every Stage of Your Life*, (New York: C.P. Putnam's Sons, 2001).

26   Bradley J. Willcox, D. Craig Willcox, and Makoto Suzuki, *The Okinawa Program*, (New York: Three Rivers Press, 2001).

27   J. David Curb et. al, "Effective Aging: Meeting the Challenge of Growing Older," in *Journal of the American Geriatrics Society*, July, 1990, Vol. 38, No. 7, pp.827–828.

28   C.G. Jung, *Psychological Types*, CW, Vol 6, par. 204. p. 126.

29   William S. Howell, *The Empathic Communicator*, (Prospect Heights, IL: Waveland Press, Inc. 1982), pp. 29–33.

30   See Riso, *Personality Types*, and Riso and Hudson, *The Wisdom of the Enneagram*.

31   See the description of the Type One on the RHETI and the detailed discussion in, Riso, *Personality Types*, pp. 376–409.

32   See the description of the Type Two on the RHETI and the detailed discussion in, Riso, *Personality Types*, pp. 59–94.

33   See the description of the Type Three on the RHETI and the detailed discussion in, Riso, *Personality Types*, pp. 95–133.

34   See the description of the Type Four on the RHETI and the detailed discussion in, Riso, *Personality Types*, pp. 134–172.

35   See the description of the Type Five on the RHETI and the detailed discussion in, Riso, *Personality Types*, pp. 173–215.

36   See the description of the Type Six on the RHETI and the detailed discussion in, Riso, *Personality Types*, pp. 216–258.

37   See the description of the Type Seven on the RHETI and the detailed discussion in, Riso, *Personality Types*, pp. 259–296.

38   See the description of the Type Eight on the RHETI and the detailed discussion in, Riso, *Personality Types*, pp. 297–337.

39   See the description of the Type Nine on the RHETI and the detailed discussion in, Riso, *Personality Types*, pp. 338–375.

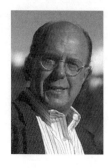

MARK BODNARCZUK is president of the Breckenridge Consulting Group Inc. and adjunct faculty member at Colorado Mountain College. Mark has a BA from Mid-America Nazarene University in religious studies, an MA from Wheaton College in theological studies, and an MA from the University of Chicago in the philosophy of science.

Mark is a personal coach, consultant, facilitator, and teacher with more than twenty years of experience working with companies in the areas of high-tech, basic and applied research, pharmaceuticals, healthcare, retail, as well as government and non-profit organizations. He has also published widely in the fields of organizational and leadership development. He is an instructor for the Enneagram and the Myers-Briggs Personality Type Indicator, and has trained over twelve hundred people in Stephen Covey's 7 Habits of Highly Effective People and Franklin-Covey's What Matters Most time management.

Mark was trained in the Enneagram by Don Richard Riso and Russ Hudson and is a professional level member of the International Enneagram Association. He has spent over eighteen years in analysis with a Jungian analyst, has recorded more than one thousand dreams over a twenty-three year period, and facilitates the process of dream interpretation for himself and others. He is a member of the C.G. Jung Institute in Denver and participates in an on-going study group on Jungian psychology.

Mark is a PADI certified Advanced Open Water Diver and has logged over three hundred scuba dives in the past four years.

∿∿∿∿

For more information about consulting services, workshops, and products please contact:

Breckenridge Consulting Group Inc.

PO Box 5050 ♦ Breckenridge, CO 80424 ♦ 1-800-303-2554

www.breckconsulting.com ♦ www.divingin.com